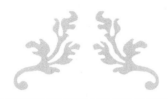

BARIATRIC COOKBOOK

*Nutritious and Delicious Recipes for Every Stage of Your Post-Surgery Journey.
Including Expert Advice and Simple Guides for Long-Term Health.*

Stefan Decker

Table of Contents

INTRODUCTION 7
    Understanding Bariatric Surgery and the Role of Nutrition 7
    Mental and Emotional Preparation for Bariatric Surgery 9
    How to Best Use the Book 10
CHAPTER 1: POST-SURGICAL NUTRITION 12
    What to Expect After Surgery 12
    Essential Macros and Micronutrients 13
    General Guidelines and Hydration 15
CHAPTER 2: PHASE 1 - LIQUID DIET 18
    Goals, duration and recommended foods 18
    Liquid Recipes 21
        1. Classic Miso Soup 21
        2. Creamy Chicken Broth 22
        3. Savory Bone Broth Elixir 22
        4. Protein-Packed Vegetable Broth 23
        5. Creamy Pumpkin Soup 23
        6. Carrot-Ginger Soup 24
        7. Smooth Cauliflower Soup 24
        8. Butternut Squash Soup 25
        9. Light Spinach and Leek Soup 25
        10. Creamy Pea Soup 26
        11. Hearty Lentil Soup 26
        12. Zesty Lemon Chicken Soup 27
        13. Silky Mushroom Soup 28
        14. Smooth Potato and Chive Soup 28
        15. Coconut Curry Broth 29
        16. Savory Egg Drop Soup 29
        17. Creamy Celery Soup 30
        18. Green Pea and Mint Soup 30
        19. Classic Gazpacho (Blended) 31
        20. Tomato Basil Soup 32
        21. Silky Zucchini Soup 32
        22. Broccoli and Cheese Soup 33
        23. Smooth Beet Soup 34
        24. Sweet Potato Coconut Soup 34
        25. Silken Tofu and Spinach Soup 35
        26. Blended Oatmeal Smoothie 35

27. Berry Protein Shake..36

28. Green Detox Shake..36

29. Peanut Butter Banana Smoothie..37

30. Creamy Chia Seed Shake...37

31. Strawberry Kefir Smoothie..38

32. Tropical Mango Smoothie..38

33. Chocolate Avocado Shake...39

34. Apple Cinnamon Protein Shake..39

35. Blueberry Almond Milk Smoothie..40

36. Iced Matcha Protein Shake...40

37. Vanilla Chai Smoothie..41

38. Cucumber Mint Cooler...41

39. Watermelon Coconut Drink..42

40. Golden Turmeric Milk..42

CHAPTER 3: PHASE 2 - SEMISOLID DIET..44

Transition and suggestions...44

Semisolid Recipes..47

41. Creamy Mashed Cauliflower..47

42. Soft Scrambled Eggs with Cheese..48

43. Smooth Cottage Cheese and Avocado Mix...48

44. Mashed Sweet Potato Delight...49

45. Silky Pumpkin Puree..49

46. Creamy Spinach and Ricotta Blend..50

47. Soft Tofu and Berry Parfait..50

48. Savory Ricotta and Herb Mash..51

49. Creamy Butternut Squash and Carrot Blend..51

50. Blended Chickpea and Tahini Puree..52

51. Creamy Lentil Mash with Herbs...52

52. Smooth Apple-Cinnamon Oatmeal...53

53. Greek Yogurt and Honey Swirl...53

54. Mango Chia Seed Pudding..54

55. Silky Carrot and Ginger Mash..54

56. Mashed Avocado with Soft-Boiled Egg..55

57. Soft Banana and Greek Yogurt Blend...56

58. Ricotta and Spinach Puree...56

59. Soft Pea and Mint Mash...57

60. Silken Tofu with Honey and Vanilla..57

61. Smooth Sweet Potato and Cinnamon Mix...58

62. Blended Chicken and Broccoli Mash...58

63. Creamy Polenta with Parmesan...59

64. Mashed Cauliflower and Cheddar Blend..60

65. Soft Baked Apple and Cinnamon Mix...60

66. Creamy Pumpkin and Quinoa Mash...61

67. Mashed Black Beans and Avocado..61

68. Smooth Zucchini and Potato Blend 62

69. Soft Cottage Cheese with Peaches 62

70. Creamy Rice Pudding with Nutmeg 63

CHAPTER 4: PHASE 3 - SOLID DIET 64

Reinsert solid foods gradually 64

Solid Recipes 67

71. Soft Grilled Chicken Strips with Herbs 67

72. Baked Salmon with Lemon and Dill 68

73. Tender Turkey Meatballs in Tomato Sauce 68

74. Soft Baked Cod with Garlic and Parsley 69

75. Creamy Chicken Salad with Greek Yogurt 69

76. Stir-Fried Tofu with Soft Vegetables 70

77. Avocado and Soft-Boiled Egg Salad 70

78. Zucchini Noodles with Marinara Sauce 71

79. Soft Baked Eggplant with Tomato and Cheese 71

80. Chicken and Avocado Lettuce Wraps 72

81. Tender Turkey and Spinach Patties 73

82. Soft Quinoa Salad with Avocado and Peas 73

83. Mashed Chickpea and Veggie Bowl 74

84. Oven-Baked Tilapia with Herbs 74

85. Soft Cauliflower Rice Stir-Fry 75

86. Baked Sweet Potato with Cottage Cheese 75

87. Creamy Tuna Salad with Soft Veggies 76

88. Soft Turkey and Vegetable Skillet 76

89. Mashed Bean and Avocado Tacos 77

90. Grilled Salmon with Mango Salsa 78

91. Soft Baked Chicken and Zucchini Casserole 78

92. Quinoa and Soft Veggie Stuffed Peppers 79

93. Soft Spinach and Cheese Stuffed Chicken 80

94. Baked Cod with Spinach and Lemon 80

95. Tender Turkey Chili 81

96. Soft Chicken and Cauliflower Bowl 81

97. Creamy Lentil and Spinach Salad 82

98. Avocado and Cucumber Sushi Rolls 82

99. Soft Quinoa and Bean Stuffed Tomatoes 83

100. Grilled Shrimp with Avocado and Mango 83

101. Soft Turkey Meatloaf with Carrots 84

102. Eggplant and Chicken Parmesan Bake 84

103. Baked Chicken with Soft Asparagus 85

104. Soft Baked Tofu and Veggie Stir-Fry 85

105. Creamy Spinach and Mushroom Omelette 86

CHAPTER 5: MAINTAINING A HEALTHY LIFESTYLE 87

Meal Planning and Managing Cravings 87

Physical Activity and Long-Term Weight Management 89

The Role of Sleep and Stress Management 90

CHAPTER 6: ADDITIONAL RESOURCES 93

Shopping Lists 93

28-Day Meal Plan 95

CONCLUSION 98

Final Reflections and Supporting Resources 98

Celebrating Milestones and Progress 100

Staying Motivated for Lifelong Success 101

BONUS 103

INTRODUCTION

---◆---

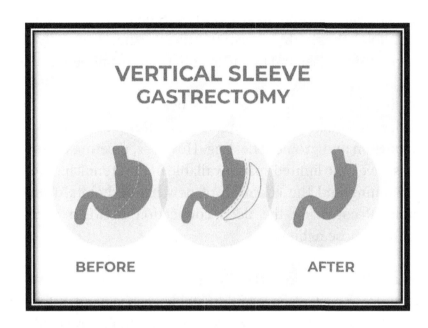

Embarking on the journey after bariatric surgery is both a challenging and rewarding experience. It's a time of transformation, where food becomes more than just sustenance, it becomes a key part of healing and health. This book is here to guide you through that journey, providing the knowledge, tools and recipes you need to nourish your body effectively. Each stage of recovery brings unique nutritional needs and understanding how to adapt your eating habits is crucial. Whether you're new to cooking or simply seeking inspiration, these pages will help you navigate your new lifestyle with confidence and care.

Understanding Bariatric Surgery and the Role of Nutrition

Bariatric surgery is more than just a medical procedure; it's a transformative journey that reshapes not just the body but the way one interacts with food and nutrition. For many, the decision to undergo this surgery marks a significant turning point, often made after years of struggling with weight management. While the surgery itself can be a powerful tool for change, its long-term success largely hinges on how well individuals adapt their eating habits to support their new physiology.

When the stomach is surgically reduced in size, it changes how much food a person can comfortably consume. More importantly, it alters how the body absorbs nutrients, making a mindful, strategic approach to nutrition essential. The newly-sized stomach requires nutrient-dense foods in smaller quantities to ensure the body gets what it needs without causing discomfort or digestive issues. Nutrition, therefore, becomes not just important, but central to this new lifestyle. The food choices made and the way meals are consumed directly impact how a person feels, heals and sustains long-term health goals.

Bariatric surgery comes with a new set of responsibilities when it comes to eating. In the past, eating might have been an automatic, sometimes mindless act. After surgery, however, it transforms into an exercise in patience, awareness and continuous learning. It's necessary to pay close attention to portion sizes, nutrient content and food textures. Small changes, like sipping water instead of gulping or chewing food thoroughly, become crucial aspects of daily life. Success is not solely determined by the procedure itself but by the ongoing commitment to a new way of eating and living.

Nutrition plays a pivotal role because the body's needs remain just as high as before, despite the reduced stomach size. Protein, vitamins, minerals and fluids are still necessary to maintain energy, support immune function and promote healing. However, meeting these nutritional needs requires a deliberate process, given the limited space available in the stomach. The smaller capacity demands thoughtful meal planning and the adoption of new eating habits, which is where this guidance becomes invaluable. Recognizing the deep connection between surgery and nutrition is the cornerstone of building those habits.

Bariatric surgery fundamentally alters the digestive process and different types of surgery, whether it's a gastric bypass, sleeve gastrectomy or adjustable gastric band, affect the body in unique ways. In some instances, the stomach is reduced to a small pouch, drastically limiting food intake. In others, parts of the intestine are bypassed, reducing calorie and nutrient absorption. This makes the choice of foods even more critical. Every meal becomes an opportunity to nourish the body effectively. Opting for foods with low nutritional value not only risks malnutrition but can also cause discomfort and potential complications.

Adjusting to this new lifestyle can be challenging and that's a completely normal part of the process. Many individuals experience a period of trial and error as they discover which foods their body tolerates best. It's common to find that certain foods, especially those high in sugar or fat, may cause digestive discomfort. Others might realize they need to focus on foods rich in protein and vitamins to meet daily requirements. This journey is about finding a balance that works, emphasizing the importance of nutritious, satisfying options that align with these new dietary needs.

Hydration is another key factor in this new nutritional landscape. The smaller stomach makes it harder to consume large quantities of fluid at once, yet staying hydrated is crucial for overall health. Sipping fluids throughout the day, rather than drinking large amounts in one sitting and avoiding liquids during meals to prevent overfilling the stomach are new habits to develop. Incorporating water-rich foods into the diet can also help maintain hydration levels without overwhelming the stomach's capacity.

Nutrition after bariatric surgery involves more than just the choice of food; it's also about the entire eating process. Slowing down, savoring each bite and listening to the body's signals of fullness become essential practices. These changes not only support physical health but also contribute to building a more positive relationship with food. Instead of seeing eating as a challenge, it can become a moment for nourishment and self-care.

The road to finding balance is filled with learning and adaptation. There will be moments of adjustment, but each step forward brings greater insight into how to fuel the body in a way that is both satisfying and healthful. This understanding forms the basis for a smoother, more successful transition into a healthy post-surgery lifestyle, where food is no longer the enemy but a valuable ally.

Mental and Emotional Preparation for Bariatric Surgery

The journey following bariatric surgery involves profound shifts not only in physical habits but also in emotional and mental perspectives. For many, food has served as more than just nourishment; it has been a source of comfort, celebration or even stress relief. This new chapter invites a re-evaluation of that relationship, moving from seeing food as a solution for emotional needs to viewing it as a way to nourish and support the body's recovery and health. This shift can bring about a wide range of emotions, some days filled with pride and joy at achieving personal milestones and others marked by frustration or a sense of loss as old habits are left behind.

Emotional adjustments can be one of the most challenging aspects of life after bariatric surgery. It's natural to feel a sense of disorientation as former ways of coping are no longer available in the same form. Eating less or making different food choices may leave one feeling deprived or nostalgic for past routines, especially during moments of stress or social gatherings. Being mindful of these feelings and acknowledging them without judgment can be a powerful step in the process. This journey encourages the discovery of new ways to nurture emotional well-being beyond food, such as connecting with supportive friends or engaging in activities that bring joy and relaxation. Journaling, talking with a counselor or simply setting aside time to reflect on the changes can help in making peace with the new eating habits and viewing them as acts of self-care.

Mentally adjusting to a new body and eating style is equally significant. As weight changes, body image may shift, leading to new self-perceptions. The mirror may reflect a smaller frame, yet mentally adjusting to these changes takes time and patience. There can be moments of uncertainty and it's common to feel a mixture of excitement and anxiety as the body transforms. Accepting these evolving changes is an essential part of the journey and celebrating each small victory can help foster a positive mindset. It's also valuable to remember that progress isn't solely defined by physical changes but by the increased sense of empowerment that comes from making mindful choices and cultivating resilience.

Social situations may also feel different after surgery. Dining out, attending gatherings or even eating with family can present unique challenges as old routines are replaced by new habits.

Explaining dietary changes or navigating questions from others can sometimes feel overwhelming. However, this is an opportunity to communicate openly about personal goals and boundaries. Setting expectations and preparing mentally for these occasions can make the experience smoother and less stressful. Over time, these situations may serve as reminders of the personal growth achieved along the way.

At the core of these mental and emotional adjustments is the realization that food, while important, is just one aspect of well-being. By shifting focus towards overall health, self-compassion and balance, the journey after bariatric surgery becomes one of self-discovery. This transformation may be challenging at times, but it's a testament to resilience and the commitment to a healthier, more fulfilling life. Each emotional challenge becomes a stepping stone, shaping a new way of being that honors both physical needs and emotional well-being. The path may not always be easy, but with each step, it leads toward a life where health, balance and self-care come together as powerful allies.

How to Best Use the Book

This book is designed to be more than just a collection of recipes; it's a guide, a companion for those navigating life after bariatric surgery. To get the most out of it, consider it a roadmap that aligns with your journey toward a healthier lifestyle. Each page is crafted to support the changes you're experiencing, providing tools and insights to help you nourish your body effectively. This isn't a one-size-fits-all guide but a tailored approach to suit the unique challenges and milestones of living post-surgery.

Begin by taking some time to explore the structure of the book. Each part corresponds to different stages of recovery and lifestyle adaptation. The recipes have been carefully created with the post-bariatric diet in mind, ensuring they meet the nutritional requirements of someone with a smaller stomach capacity while still being enjoyable. They offer a balance of flavors, textures and nutrients that work together to promote healing, sustain energy and support weight management. The goal is not just to survive on a limited diet, but to thrive within it.

There's no rush to jump from one phase to the next. This book encourages a gradual approach, respecting the body's pace. Listen to your body, observe how it responds to different foods and use that feedback as your guide. The progression of recipes is meant to walk you through each step, moving from liquids to semisolids and eventually to more solid foods. Treat each section as a foundation to build upon, giving your digestive system the time it needs to adapt. If you find yourself struggling with a particular food or texture, revisit earlier sections and experiment until you're comfortable. This process is about honoring your body's signals and finding what works best for you.

Cooking after bariatric surgery requires some mindfulness and planning, but that doesn't mean it has to be a chore. The recipes here are intended to make the process enjoyable, introducing you to new ways of thinking about food. Focus on quality over quantity. You're now looking at smaller portions, so the importance of each ingredient grows. Use this opportunity to explore new flavors, try different spices and discover meals that not only meet your dietary needs but also bring joy to the table. Eating post-surgery is an experience that can and should be pleasurable, even with the necessary adjustments.

When you approach the recipes, keep an open mind. You may encounter dishes that feel unfamiliar or ingredients you haven't used before. That's part of the journey. Each recipe includes detailed instructions to help you navigate preparation, cooking and serving with ease. Start with what feels comfortable, then gradually explore other recipes as you grow more confident. If you've never used something like tofu or quinoa before, think of this as a chance to expand your culinary horizons in a way that supports your health goals. Remember, there is no right or wrong way to experience these recipes, only the way that works for you.

It's also important to pay attention to how you eat, not just what you eat. Bariatric surgery changes your relationship with food and this book is here to guide you through that new dynamic. As you try different recipes, notice how they make you feel. Are you satisfied? Are you full but not uncomfortable? Use those experiences to fine-tune your choices. If you're still hungry after a meal, consider if it was due to the texture, flavor or portion size. This process is as much about learning to listen to your body's cues as it is about following a recipe.

Beyond the recipes, this book provides insights into the types of foods that work best during each phase. Think of it as a toolkit for your journey, equipping you with knowledge and options to make mealtime easier. The goal is to empower you to take control of your eating habits and develop a routine that fits your lifestyle. Cooking becomes not just a means to an end but an act of self-care, a moment where you can connect with your new way of living and embrace the changes.

Feel free to adapt the recipes to suit your taste preferences and dietary needs. Swap ingredients if certain foods don't sit well with you, adjust seasonings to match your palate and take creative liberties to make each dish truly yours. The recipes are not set in stone but rather serve as a starting point for your culinary exploration. Cooking after bariatric surgery is about flexibility, adaptability and learning to nourish your body in a way that feels right for you.

Use this book as your kitchen ally, a source of inspiration and guidance. Allow it to support you through the ups and downs of this journey, providing a steady, reliable resource whenever you need it. With each recipe, you're not just preparing a meal; you're building a lifestyle that aligns with your health and well-being. Take it one step at a time and remember that each small change adds up to a meaningful transformation.

Chapter 1: Post-Surgical Nutrition

---------- ❖ ----------

The period following bariatric surgery is a time of immense change, especially when it comes to nutrition. Your body now functions differently and understanding how to meet its new needs is essential for recovery and long-term success. This phase is about learning what your body can handle, choosing foods that provide maximum nourishment in smaller quantities and developing mindful eating habits. By focusing on the right balance of nutrients, hydration and meal practices you set the foundation for a healthier, more manageable lifestyle that aligns with your new reality.

What to Expect After Surgery

The days and weeks following bariatric surgery are a whirlwind of changes, not just physically but mentally and emotionally as well. As you wake up from the procedure, the first thing you'll notice is that your body feels different. There's a sensation of fullness in your abdomen and your stomach now much smaller, sends new signals. You'll need to take things slowly, allowing your body to begin the healing process. This period is about listening to these new cues and understanding how your body has changed.

During the initial days post-surgery, you'll likely experience some discomfort. It's normal to feel bloated, with occasional cramping or nausea as your digestive system adjusts. Your healthcare team will provide guidance on managing these feelings, often recommending that you start with small sips of water or clear broth. Hydration becomes a critical focus from the very beginning, as your body needs fluids to recover and flush out the anesthesia and medications used during surgery. Remember, your new stomach can only hold a few ounces at a time, so taking tiny sips is key. Gulping down large amounts, which might have been second nature before, will now lead to discomfort and even vomiting. This is the first glimpse of the mindful eating practices that will shape your new relationship with food.

The immediate aftermath of surgery also brings a temporary, yet profound change in your appetite. For many, the constant feeling of hunger diminishes, replaced by a sense of fullness even after consuming very little. This is your body's way of adjusting to its new normal, as hormones involved in hunger regulation shift. This change can be liberating but also requires a recalibration of your eating habits.

What once might have been automatic, like grabbing a snack when feeling peckish, now demands conscious thought and planning. You'll notice that eating is no longer about volume; it's about choosing foods that truly nourish you in small, satisfying amounts.

Your taste preferences might also take an unexpected turn. Foods you once craved may now seem too rich, too sweet or even unappealing. This change is a common side effect of the surgery, often driven by both the physical alterations to your digestive system and the new awareness you develop around what you consume. These shifts are an opportunity to explore new flavors and textures that align with your body's changing needs. However, it's important to introduce foods cautiously. Your stomach is healing and pushing the boundaries too soon can lead to discomfort or setbacks.

Emotionally, this phase can be both exciting and daunting. The rapid physical changes, combined with the new rules around eating, can feel overwhelming. Many people experience a mix of emotions, ranging from hope and pride to frustration and anxiety. This is entirely normal. You're not just learning how to eat differently; you're redefining your relationship with food and your body. Some days will feel easier than others and that's okay. What matters is approaching each day with patience and compassion for yourself as you adapt to this new way of living.

In this early stage, rest is as crucial as nutrition. Your body has undergone a major surgery and it needs time to heal. Physical activity, while beneficial, will be limited to gentle movements such as short walks. This isn't the time to push for exercise goals; it's about getting your body moving just enough to promote circulation and prevent complications. Similarly, you'll be focusing on liquid intake for nourishment.

Your meals will be limited to clear liquids and broth, progressing to protein shakes and pureed foods as your stomach begins to tolerate more variety. This liquid phase is a fundamental part of the recovery process, giving your digestive system time to adjust to its new structure.

As you navigate these first days and weeks, the most important thing to remember is that this is just the beginning of your journey. Your body is working hard to adapt and heal and it will take some time before you find a new rhythm. Trust the process, listen to your body's signals and lean on the support of your healthcare team and loved ones. There will be moments of discomfort, confusion and uncertainty, but there will also be moments of joy as you discover what your new lifestyle makes possible.

Understanding what to expect after surgery helps set the foundation for the changes to come. This period is about laying down new habits, learning to recognize and respect the signals from your body and beginning the process of nourishing yourself in a way that supports your health goals. There's no right or wrong way to feel during this time; it's a unique experience for everyone. What matters is that you give yourself the space and patience to adjust to this new chapter in your life.

ESSENTIAL MACROS AND MICRONUTRIENTS

Post-surgery, nutrition takes on a whole new meaning. Your body has undergone a major change and the nutrients you consume will play a pivotal role in your recovery and overall health. With your stomach now holding significantly less food, every bite counts. The focus shifts from simply eating to choosing foods that provide maximum nutrition in small quantities. This is where the importance of macronutrients and micronutrients comes into sharp focus. Knowing what your body needs and why can help you make smarter food choices that support your healing process and long-term well-being.

Protein is the superstar of post-bariatric nutrition. After surgery, your body needs protein to heal and maintain muscle mass. Muscle loss can be a concern with rapid weight reduction, so prioritizing protein intake is key. Since your meals are now much smaller, it's crucial to include a source of high-quality protein in every meal. Lean meats like chicken or turkey, fish, eggs, low-fat dairy products, tofu and protein shakes become your go-to options. Unlike before, when protein might have been just another part of the plate, it now takes center stage.Consuming enough protein helps with satiety, keeps energy levels steady and aids in the recovery of tissues. In those early weeks of recovery, even small amounts of protein can make a big difference. For example, a few spoonfuls of cottage cheese or a half cup of Greek yogurt can provide the protein your body craves in a form that's easy to digest.

While protein often steals the spotlight, carbohydrates and fats are still vital. However, they require a more mindful approach. After surgery, the types of carbohydrates you consume should be primarily complex, like those found in vegetables, legumes and whole grains. These carbs digest more slowly, helping to maintain stable blood sugar levels and providing a steady source of energy. Refined carbs and sugars, which can cause rapid spikes and drops in blood sugar, become less friendly to your new digestive system. Not to mention, they often don't offer the nutritional benefits that your body needs most. Think of complex carbs as fuel for your day, especially when combined with fiber-rich vegetables that support digestion and add bulk to your meals, helping you feel satisfied.

Fats are equally essential, but the focus shifts to healthier sources like avocados, nuts, seeds and olive oil. These fats support cell structure, hormone production and nutrient absorption. However, given the smaller stomach size and the potential for digestive sensitivity, fats should be consumed in moderation. They are calorie-dense, which means even small amounts can provide the necessary energy without taking up too much room. A drizzle of olive oil over a salad, a spoonful of nut butter or a few slices of avocado are all examples of ways to incorporate healthy fats into your meals without overwhelming your stomach.

Micronutrients, though needed in smaller quantities, are just as crucial. After bariatric surgery, the risk of vitamin and mineral deficiencies increases due to the reduced food intake and, in some cases, changes in how the digestive system absorbs nutrients. Vitamins and minerals like iron, calcium, vitamin D, B12 and folate become priorities. They support everything from bone health to immune function to energy production. While a well-balanced diet can provide many of these nutrients, your healthcare provider may recommend supplements to ensure you're getting enough.

Iron, for example, can be challenging to absorb after certain types of bariatric surgery. Iron-rich foods like lean meats, beans and spinach can help, but even these might not be enough to meet your body's needs. Vitamin B12 also deserves special attention, as it requires a specific part of the stomach for absorption, which may have been altered by surgery. Foods like eggs, dairy and fortified cereals can contribute to your B12 intake, but supplementation is often necessary to maintain adequate levels.

Calcium and vitamin D work hand in hand to support bone health. With a limited capacity to consume dairy products and other calcium-rich foods, a daily calcium supplement often becomes part of the routine. Pairing it with vitamin D ensures your body can properly absorb and use the calcium you're taking in. Magnesium, zinc and other trace minerals also contribute to the body's overall functioning, even though they're needed in much smaller amounts.

Hydration, while technically not a macronutrient or micronutrient, plays a supporting role in nutrient absorption and digestion. Dehydration can exacerbate feelings of fatigue and slow the body's recovery. Sipping water throughout the day, instead of drinking large quantities all at once, helps keep your body hydrated and supports its ability to process the nutrients you consume.

Understanding the roles these nutrients play and how to include them in your new dietary routine sets the stage for a successful post-surgical lifestyle. Each bite, each choice you make, is an opportunity to fuel your body in a way that aligns with your health goals. It's about finding balance, choosing nutrient-dense options and giving your body the support it needs to thrive.

General Guidelines and Hydration

Adjusting to life after bariatric surgery requires a new set of eating habits and practices. The changes made to your digestive system mean that meals, portions and even the act of drinking fluids need to be approached with care and mindfulness. These guidelines are not mere rules but tools to help you get the most out of your new lifestyle. They guide you through the early stages of recovery and become the foundation of your eating habits going forward.

One of the first adjustments is embracing smaller, more frequent meals. After surgery, your stomach can hold only a small amount of food at one time, so it's important to focus on eating multiple small meals throughout the day. This not only helps you meet your nutritional needs but also prevents discomfort and overstretching of the stomach pouch. It's a process of learning to eat slowly and to stop when you feel satisfied, not full. Each meal should be consumed slowly, giving your body time to signal when it's had enough.

Eating too quickly or taking large bites can lead to nausea or discomfort. Chewing food thoroughly becomes essential, breaking it down to a soft consistency that's easier for your stomach to handle. This is a major shift from how many of us are used to eating, especially in a world where meals are often rushed. It requires patience and a commitment to listening to your body's signals, turning each meal into a mindful experience.

Portion control takes on a whole new meaning post-surgery. With your stomach's reduced size, it's important to start with smaller amounts and adjust based on how your body responds. Your eyes may still crave the large portions you were once used to, but now it's about retraining your mindset. Using smaller plates, bowls and utensils can help. They make smaller portions appear more substantial and encourage slower, more mindful eating. Measuring out food in the beginning can also help you gauge what a serving size looks like. Over time, you'll become more attuned to recognizing the right amount without the need to measure everything.

The timing of meals is another important aspect. Spacing out your meals throughout the day – typically three small meals with one or two healthy snacks – allows your body to digest food effectively without feeling overwhelmed. Avoiding distractions during meals is also beneficial. Eating in front of the TV or while scrolling through your phone can make it harder to listen to your body's signals, leading to overeating or discomfort. Making meals a dedicated time for nourishment and self-care will support your transition into this new lifestyle.

Hydration plays a crucial role in your recovery and overall health. After bariatric surgery, staying hydrated can be more challenging due to the reduced capacity of your stomach. The key is to sip fluids throughout the day rather than drinking large quantities at once. It may sound simple, but it's a habit that takes time to master. A common guideline is to aim for at least 64 ounces of fluids daily, though individual needs can vary. Water is the best choice, but other non-carbonated, sugar-free beverages can also contribute to your hydration.

It's important to separate drinking from eating. Before surgery, having a beverage with a meal might have been second nature. However, after surgery, drinking while eating can lead to discomfort and push food through your stomach too quickly, which can hinder the feeling of fullness. To avoid this, it's recommended to stop drinking fluids at least 30 minutes before a meal and to wait about 30 minutes after eating before you start sipping again. This might feel unnatural at first, but it becomes easier as you develop a new rhythm. The goal is to allow food to settle in your stomach, providing you with the sensation of satiety without interference from liquids.

Carbonated drinks are best avoided, as they can introduce gas into your stomach and cause bloating or discomfort. Caffeine and alcohol also need to be approached with caution. Caffeine, found in coffee, tea and some sodas, can irritate the stomach lining and may affect hydration. If you choose to reintroduce caffeine into your diet, it's advisable to do so slowly and in moderation, paying attention to how your body reacts. Alcohol poses its own set of challenges. Not only can it be harsh on your stomach, but its effects are often intensified after bariatric surgery. If you decide to drink alcohol, it should be done sparingly and with full awareness of its stronger impact.

Hydration isn't just about drinking fluids; it's about incorporating water-rich foods into your diet as well. Foods like cucumbers, watermelon and leafy greens can provide both hydration and nutrients. Soups and broths are also great options, especially in the earlier stages when you're limited to a more liquid-based diet. These foods serve as an additional source of fluid intake, complementing your daily water consumption.

Navigating post-surgical nutrition is about embracing new habits and listening to your body's signals. It's a journey of rediscovery, exploring how to eat, what to eat and how to stay hydrated in ways that support your well-being. These changes are more than temporary adjustments; they're the building blocks for a lasting lifestyle that prioritizes your health. By being mindful, patient and informed, you empower yourself to thrive with a diet that nurtures both body and spirit.

Chapter 2: Phase 1 - Liquid Diet

———— ❖ ————

The liquid diet phase marks the first crucial step in your post-surgery recovery. This period is all about giving your stomach the rest it needs while beginning to nourish your body in a new way. The foods you choose now should be gentle, nutrient-rich and easy to digest, helping to kickstart the healing process. It's a time to focus on sipping slowly, listening to your body's signals and embracing small, intentional meals. While this phase may feel restrictive, it lays the groundwork for a successful transition into your new eating habits and lifestyle.

Goals, duration and recommended foods

The liquid diet phase is the first step in your post-surgical journey, setting the tone for your recovery and helping your body adjust to its new way of processing food. It might seem restrictive at first, but it serves a vital purpose. The goal of this phase is to allow your stomach to heal while gently reintroducing nourishment. During this time, your digestive system needs to rest and recover from the surgery. By consuming only liquids, you minimize the risk of irritation or strain on your newly adjusted stomach, which is crucial for avoiding complications and ensuring a smooth healing process.

This phase is not just about what you're consuming but also about relearning how to consume. Your body is now sending different signals and it's essential to pay attention to them. The sensation of hunger will change, as will the feeling of fullness. Sipping slowly, taking breaks and noticing how your body responds to each intake of liquid are new habits that you'll start developing now. It's about resetting your approach to nourishment, with the focus on gentle, mindful consumption.

The liquid diet typically lasts for about one to two weeks, depending on your surgeon's advice and how your body is responding. It's important to be patient during this time. While it might feel challenging, this phase is temporary and is designed to give you the best possible start to your new lifestyle. Rushing through it or introducing solid foods too soon can put unnecessary stress on your stomach and may slow down your recovery. Trust the process and use this time to explore a variety of liquid options that not only meet your nutritional needs but also help you adapt to this new way of eating.

When we talk about recommended foods during the liquid phase, it's more than just basic hydration. The liquids you consume need to be packed with nutrients to support healing, maintain energy and set the groundwork for healthy eating habits moving forward. Water is, of course, essential. Staying hydrated helps flush out toxins and supports every function of your body. However, plain water alone will not provide the nutrients your body needs. This is where nutrient-rich liquids come into play.

Broths are a staple during this phase, offering both hydration and some level of nourishment. Bone broth, in particular, is rich in minerals like calcium, magnesium and phosphorus and provides collagen, which is beneficial for tissue repair. A warm, savory broth can be soothing, especially when your stomach is still sensitive. Vegetable and chicken broths are also great options, providing a subtle flavor while being gentle on your digestive system.

Protein is another key player during the liquid phase. Your body is in the midst of healing and protein is the building block for repairing tissues and maintaining muscle mass. Protein shakes or drinks become a daily requirement to meet your body's needs. Look for high-quality, low-sugar options, preferably those that are specifically formulated for post-bariatric patients. These shakes can be mixed with water, unsweetened almond milk or other liquid bases to create a satisfying, nutrient-dense beverage. When choosing protein supplements, aim for those that offer at least 15 to 20 grams of protein per serving. This will help you meet your daily protein goals, which are critical in this phase and beyond.

Smooth, blended soups are another way to introduce variety while sticking to the liquid requirement. Puree vegetables like carrots, zucchini and butternut squash with a bit of broth to create a creamy texture that's easy to sip. The natural sweetness and nutrients in these vegetables provide not just flavor but also vitamins and minerals that aid in recovery. These soups should be strained to remove any small bits of fiber or solids that might irritate your stomach. Adding a small amount of unflavored protein powder to these soups can boost their nutritional content, ensuring you're getting both the taste and the nourishment your body craves.

Milk and dairy alternatives, like unsweetened almond or soy milk, can be used as bases for protein shakes or consumed on their own. They offer additional protein and calcium, supporting bone health and muscle maintenance. Some people find comfort in sipping warm milk with a dash of vanilla extract or cinnamon, creating a soothing, nutritious drink. However, it's important to listen to your body; some individuals may have temporary lactose intolerance post-surgery, so plant-based milk options are great alternatives.

Sugar-free gelatin and popsicles can add a bit of variety and are often welcomed during this period of liquid-only intake. They offer a change in texture and temperature, which can make the diet feel less monotonous. However, these should be consumed in moderation, as they don't provide significant nutritional value. The main focus should remain on nutrient-dense liquids that support your body's healing process.

Sipping on electrolyte-infused drinks can also help maintain your body's mineral balance, especially if you're feeling lightheaded or fatigued. Post-surgery, your body might be prone to dehydration, so finding ways to maintain electrolyte levels is crucial. Opt for sugar-free versions to avoid unnecessary calories and consider coconut water as a natural alternative, though in small amounts due to its natural sugar content.

The liquid phase is a time to embrace simplicity while focusing on nourishment. It's less about taste and more about function. These liquids serve as the foundation upon which you'll build more complex eating habits in the future. Learning to sip slowly and being mindful of how different liquids make you feel helps you tune in to your body's signals. This is the beginning of a new way of eating, one that emphasizes nutrition, patience and the understanding that each choice is a step toward a healthier you.

Liquid Recipes

❖

1. Classic Miso Soup

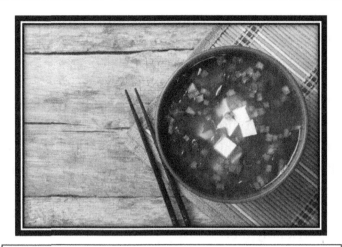

🔪 5 Min. 🕐 10 Min. 🍲 2 Serv. ⚱ Easy

Ingredients:
- 2 cups water
- 2 tbsp miso paste
- 1/4 cup silken tofu, cubed
- 1/4 tsp dashi powder
- 1 green onion, finely sliced

Preparation:
1. In a pot, bring water to a simmer. Add the dashi powder and stir.
2. Add the miso paste, stirring until completely dissolved.
3. Add the tofu cubes and simmer for 5 minutes.
4. Garnish with green onions before serving.

Comment: This light and flavorful soup is both quick to prepare and packed with authentic taste. Perfect for a balanced diet, it offers a boost of light protein with minimal effort.

Nutritional info (per serving): Cal 250 | Carb 18g | Fat 18g | Prot 5g | Fib 5g.

2. Creamy Chicken Broth

> ✎ 5 Min.   ⏱ 20 Min.   🍲 2 Serv.   👨‍🍳 Easy

Ingredients:

- 2 cups low-sodium chicken broth
- 1/4 cup plain Greek yogurt
- 1 clove garlic, minced
- 1/4 tsp onion powder
- Salt and pepper to taste

Preparation:

1. In a pot, bring the chicken broth to a simmer over medium heat.
2. Add the minced garlic and onion powder, stirring well.
3. Remove the pot from heat. Add the Greek yogurt and stir until fully combined and smooth.
4. Return to low heat for 2 minutes, but do not let it boil. Season with salt and pepper to taste.

Comment: Creamy yet light, this broth is packed with protein and made in just minutes. A soothing option for your bariatric-friendly diet.

Nutritional info (per serving): Cal 70 | Carb 2g | Fat 2g | Prot 10g | Fib 0g.

3. Savory Bone Broth Elixir

> ✎ 5 Min.   ⏱ 15 Min.   🍲 2 Serv.   👨‍🍳 Easy

Ingredients:

- 2 cups bone broth
- 1 tbsp apple cider vinegar
- 1/4 tsp turmeric powder
- 1/4 tsp black pepper
- 1/2 tsp ginger, grated

Preparation:

1. Heat the bone broth in a pot over medium heat.
2. Add the apple cider vinegar, turmeric, black pepper and grated ginger.
3. Stir well and simmer for 10 minutes. Serve hot.

Comment: This aromatic elixir combines rich flavors with the anti-inflammatory benefits o turmeric and ginger. A nourishing choice to warm you up.

Nutritional info (per serving): Cal 40 | Carb 2g | Fat 0g | Prot 8g | Fib 0g.

4. Protein-Packed Vegetable Broth

🔪 5 Min. 🕐 20 Min. 🍽 2 Serv. 👨‍🍳 Easy

Ingredients:
- 2 cups vegetable broth
- 1/4 cup unflavored protein powder
- 1 tbsp soy sauce
- 1/4 tsp garlic powder
- 1/4 tsp smoked paprika

Preparation:
1. In a pot, bring the vegetable broth to a simmer.
2. Gradually whisk in the protein powder until fully dissolved.
3. Add soy sauce, garlic powder and smoked paprika. Stir well.
4. Simmer for 10 minutes, then serve.

Comment: This warm and flavorful broth is enriched with protein, making it both light and satisfying. A great option for gentle nourishment.

Nutritional info (per serving): Cal 60 | Carb 4g | Fat 1g | Prot 10g | Fib 0g.

5. Creamy Pumpkin Soup

🔪 5 Min. 🕐 15 Min. 🍽 2 Serv. 👨‍🍳 Easy

Ingredients:
- 1 cup canned pumpkin puree
- 1 cup low-sodium vegetable broth
- 1/2 cup unsweetened almond milk
- 1/4 tsp nutmeg
- Salt and pepper to taste

Preparation:
1. In a pot, combine the pumpkin puree, vegetable broth and almond milk.
2. Stir in the nutmeg and bring to a gentle simmer for 10 minutes.
3. Season with salt and pepper to taste, then serve warm.

Comment: This silky pumpkin soup offers natural sweetness and comforting spices. Light and easy to digest, it's perfect for a balanced meal.

Nutritional info (per serving): Cal 80 | Carb 14g | Fat 2g | Prot 3g | Fib 2g.

6. Carrot-Ginger Soup

🔪 5 Min. 🕐 20 Min. 🍲 2 Serv. 🧑‍🍳 Easy

Ingredients:
- 2 cups low-sodium vegetable broth
- 1 cup carrots, peeled and chopped
- 1/2 tsp ginger, grated
- 1/4 cup coconut milk
- Salt and pepper to taste

Preparation:
1. In a pot, combine vegetable broth, carrots and ginger. Bring to a boil.
2. Reduce heat and simmer for 15 minutes until carrots are tender.
3. Use an immersion blender to puree the soup until smooth. Stir in coconut milk.
4. Season with salt and pepper before serving.

Comment: A delicate blend of carrot sweetness and ginger warmth, this soup provides both flavor and gentle nourishment. Ideal for light eating.

Nutritional info (per serving): Cal 90 | Carb 12g | Fat 4g | Prot 2g | Fib 3g.

7. Smooth Cauliflower Soup

🔪 5 Min. 🕐 20 Min. 🍲 2 Serv. 🧑‍🍳 Easy

Ingredients:
- 1 cup cauliflower florets
- 2 cups low-sodium chicken broth
- 1/4 cup heavy cream
- 1 garlic clove, minced
- Salt and pepper to taste

Preparation:
1. In a pot, combine cauliflower, chicken broth and garlic. Bring to a boil.
2. Reduce heat and simmer for 15 minutes until cauliflower is tender.

3. Blend the mixture until smooth. Stir in the heavy cream.
4. Season with salt and pepper to taste.

Comment: Smooth and creamy, this cauliflower soup combines a rich texture with wholesome ingredients. A perfect addition to a bariatric meal plan.

Nutritional info (per serving): Cal 100 | Carb 6g | Fat 7g | Prot 5g | Fib 2g.

8. BUTTERNUT SQUASH SOUP

> ✎ 5 Min. ⏱ 20 Min. ◉ 2 Serv. ♨ Easy

Ingredients:
- 1 cup butternut squash, peeled and cubed
- 2 cups low-sodium vegetable broth
- 1/4 cup coconut milk
- 1/4 tsp cinnamon
- Salt to taste

Preparation:
1. In a pot, combine the squash and broth. Bring to a boil.
2. Reduce heat and simmer for 15 minutes until the squash is tender.
3. Puree the mixture using an immersion blender. Stir in the coconut milk and cinnamon.
4. Season with salt before serving.

Comment: Naturally sweet and enhanced by a hint of cinnamon, this soup is both comforting and nutritious. It's a satisfying way to enjoy squash.

Nutritional info (per serving): Cal 110 | Carb 16g | Fat 5g | Prot 2g | Fib 3g.

9. LIGHT SPINACH AND LEEK SOUP

> ✎ 5 Min. ⏱ 15 Min. ◉ 2 Serv. ♨ Easy

Ingredients:
- 1 cup spinach leaves
- 1 leek, white part only, sliced
- 2 cups low-sodium chicken broth
- 1/4 cup plain Greek yogurt
- Salt and pepper to taste

Preparation:

1. In a pot, combine spinach, leeks and chicken broth. Bring to a boil.
2. Reduce heat and simmer for 10 minutes.
3. Use an immersion blender to puree the mixture. Stir in Greek yogurt.
4. Season with salt and pepper before serving.

Comment: Packed with tender greens and a light yogurt finish, this soup is gentle yet nourishing. A flavorful way to include vegetables in your diet.

Nutritional info (per serving): Cal 70 | Carb 9g | Fat 2g | Prot 6g | Fib 2g.

10. Creamy Pea Soup

> 🔪 5 Min.   🕐 15 Min.   🍲 2 Serv.   👨‍🍳 Easy

Ingredients:

- 1 cup frozen peas
- 1 cup low-sodium vegetable broth
- 1/4 cup coconut milk
- 1/4 tsp garlic powder
- Salt to taste

Preparation:

1. In a pot, combine peas and vegetable broth. Bring to a boil.
2. Reduce heat and simmer for 10 minutes until peas are tender.
3. Use an immersion blender to puree the soup. Stir in coconut milk and garlic powder.
4. Season with salt before serving.

Comment: The sweetness of peas pairs beautifully with creamy coconut milk for a light yet satisfying soup. A wholesome and delightful choice.

Nutritional info (per serving): Cal 90 | Carb 14g | Fat 3g | Prot 3g | Fib 4g.

11. Hearty Lentil Soup

> 🔪 5 Min.   🕐 20 Min.   🍲 2 Serv.   👨‍🍳 Easy

Ingredients:

- 1/2 cup red lentils, rinsed
- 2 cups low-sodium vegetable broth
- 1/4 cup carrot, finely chopped

- 1/4 tsp cumin powder
- Salt and pepper to taste

Preparation:
1. In a pot, combine lentils, broth and carrots. Bring to a boil.
2. Reduce heat and simmer for 15 minutes until lentils are tender.
3. Use an immersion blender to partially puree the soup. Stir in cumin.
4. Season with salt and pepper before serving.

Comment: Packed with plant-based protein and fiber, this hearty lentil soup is both filling and easy to prepare. Perfect for a balanced diet.

Nutritional info (per serving): Cal 130 | Carb 22g | Fat 1g | Prot 8g | Fib 4g.

12. Zesty Lemon Chicken Soup

✎ 5 Min. ⏱ 15 Min. ◎ 2 Serv. 👨‍🍳 Easy

Ingredients:
- 2 cups low-sodium chicken broth
- 1/4 cup cooked chicken breast, shredded
- 1 tbsp lemon juice
- 1/4 tsp garlic powder
- Salt and pepper to taste

Preparation:
1. In a pot, bring the chicken broth to a simmer.
2. Add shredded chicken, lemon juice and garlic powder. Stir well.
3. Simmer for 10 minutes. Season with salt and pepper to taste.

Comment: The brightness of lemon elevates this light chicken soup, making it refreshing and nourishing. A great choice for a soothing meal.

Nutritional info (per serving): Cal 80 | Carb 2g | Fat 1g | Prot 14g | Fib 0g.

13. Silky Mushroom Soup

| 🔪 5 Min. | 🕐 20 Min. | 🍲 2 Serv. | 👨‍🍳 Easy |

Ingredients:
- 1 cup mushrooms, sliced
- 2 cups low-sodium chicken broth
- 1/4 cup heavy cream
- 1/4 tsp thyme
- Salt and pepper to taste

Preparation:
1. In a pot, combine mushrooms and chicken broth. Bring to a boil.
2. Reduce heat and simmer for 15 minutes until mushrooms are tender.
3. Use an immersion blender to puree the mixture. Stir in heavy cream and thyme.
4. Season with salt and pepper before serving.

Comment: Creamy and earthy, this mushroom soup offers rich flavors with a delicate texture. A comforting option for light eating.

Nutritional info (per serving): Cal 120 | Carb 7g | Fat 9g | Prot 5g | Fib 1g.

14. Smooth Potato and Chive Soup

| 🔪 5 Min. | 🕐 20 Min. | 🍲 2 Serv. | 👨‍🍳 Easy |

Ingredients:
- 1 cup potatoes, peeled and diced
- 2 cups low-sodium vegetable broth
- 1/4 cup plain Greek yogurt
- 1 tbsp fresh chives, chopped
- Salt and pepper to taste

Preparation:
1. In a pot, combine potatoes and vegetable broth. Bring to a boil.
2. Reduce heat and simmer for 15 minutes until potatoes are tender.
3. Use an immersion blender to puree the soup. Stir in Greek yogurt and chives.
4. Season with salt and pepper before serving.

Comment: The creamy texture of this potato soup is complemented by the freshness of chives. A simple yet flavorful dish for gentle nourishment.

Nutritional info (per serving): Cal 110 | Carb 20g | Fat 2g | Prot 5g | Fib 2g.

15. Coconut Curry Broth

✎ 5 Min. 🕐 15 Min. 🍲 2 Serv. 👨‍🍳 Easy

Ingredients:
- 2 cups low-sodium vegetable broth
- 1/4 cup coconut milk
- 1/2 tsp curry powder
- 1 clove garlic, minced
- Salt to taste

Preparation:
1. In a pot, combine the vegetable broth and coconut milk. Bring to a simmer over medium heat.
2. Add the curry powder and minced garlic. Stir well.
3. Simmer for 10 minutes. Season with salt to taste before serving.

Comment: With the warmth of curry and the creaminess of coconut milk, this broth is aromatic and satisfying. A flavorful twist on a light soup.

Nutritional info (per serving): Cal 90 | Carb 8g | Fat 6g | Prot 2g | Fib 1g.

16. Savory Egg Drop Soup

✎ 5 Min. 🕐 10 Min. 🍲 2 Serv. 👨‍🍳 Easy

Ingredients:
- 2 cups low-sodium chicken broth
- 1 egg, beaten
- 1/4 tsp sesame oil
- 1/4 tsp soy sauce
- 1 green onion, finely chopped

Preparation:
1. In a pot, bring the chicken broth to a boil.
2. Reduce heat to low and slowly drizzle the beaten egg into the broth while stirring gently to create ribbons.
3. Stir in the sesame oil and soy sauce. Simmer for 2 minutes.
4. Garnish with chopped green onion before serving.

Comment: Simple yet rich in protein, this egg drop soup is comforting and easy to digest. A quick and wholesome choice for any meal.

Nutritional info (per serving): Cal 50 | Carb 1g | Fat 2g | Prot 6g | Fib 0g.

17. Creamy Celery Soup

🔪 5 Min.   🕐 20 Min.   🍽 2 Serv.   👨‍🍳 Easy

Ingredients:
- 1 cup celery, chopped
- 2 cups low-sodium vegetable broth
- 1/4 cup plain Greek yogurt
- 1 clove garlic, minced
- Salt and pepper to taste

Preparation:
1. In a pot, combine celery, vegetable broth and garlic. Bring to a boil.
2. Reduce heat and simmer for 15 minutes until celery is tender.
3. Use an immersion blender to puree the mixture. Stir in the Greek yogurt.
4. Season with salt and pepper to taste before serving.

Comment: The subtle flavor of celery shines in this creamy and light soup. A nutritious way to incorporate vegetables into your diet.

Nutritional info (per serving): Cal 60 | Carb 10g | Fat 1g | Prot 4g | Fib 1g.

18. Green Pea and Mint Soup

🔪 5 Min.   🕐 15 Min.   🍽 2 Serv.   👨‍🍳 Easy

Ingredients:
- 1 cup frozen peas
- 2 cups low-sodium vegetable broth
- 1/4 cup fresh mint leaves
- 1/4 cup coconut milk
- Salt to taste

Preparation:
1. In a pot, combine peas and vegetable broth. Bring to a boil.

2. Reduce heat and simmer for 10 minutes until peas are tender.
3. Add the fresh mint leaves and use an immersion blender to puree the soup.
4. Stir in the coconut milk. Season with salt before serving.

Comment: This refreshing pea soup is brightened with fresh mint, creating a unique and light combination. Ideal for a nourishing snack or meal.

Nutritional info (per serving): Cal 80 | Carb 12g | Fat 3g | Prot 3g | Fib 2g.

19. Classic Gazpacho (Blended)

🖊 10 Min. 🕒 0 Min. 🍲 2 Serv. 🎍 Easy

Ingredients:
- 1 cup tomatoes, chopped
- 1/2 cup cucumber, peeled and chopped
- 1/4 cup red bell pepper, chopped
- 1 tbsp olive oil
- Salt and pepper to taste

Preparation:
1. In a blender, combine tomatoes, cucumber and red bell pepper. Blend until smooth.
2. Add olive oil and blend for an additional 30 seconds.
3. Season with salt and pepper to taste. Chill in the refrigerator for 30 minutes before serving.

Comment: Cool and refreshing, this blended gazpacho is packed with fresh vegetables and vibrant flavors. A great option for a light meal or snack.

Nutritional info (per serving): Cal 90 | Carb 10g | Fat 5g | Prot 2g | Fib 2g.

20. Tomato Basil Soup

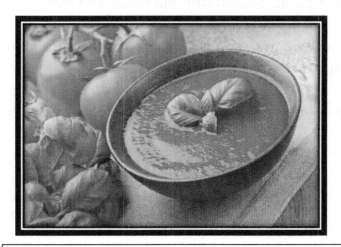

🔪 5 Min. 🕐 15 Min. 🍲 2 Serv. 👨‍🍳 Easy

Ingredients:

- 1 cup canned crushed tomatoes
- 1 cup vegetable broth
- 1/4 cup plain Greek yogurt
- 1 tsp dried basil
- Salt and pepper to taste

Preparation:

1. In a pot, combine crushed tomatoes and vegetable broth. Bring to a simmer.
2. Stir in the dried basil and simmer for 10 minutes.
3. Remove from heat and blend until smooth. Stir in Greek yogurt.
4. Season with salt and pepper before serving.

Comment: The classic combination of tomato and basil shines in this creamy soup, offering a comforting and nutritious dish. Simple yet satisfying.

Nutritional info (per serving): Cal 80 | Carb 14g | Fat 2g | Prot 4g | Fib 2g.

21. Silky Zucchini Soup

🔪 5 Min. 🕐 20 Min. 🍲 2 Serv. 👨‍🍳 Easy

Ingredients:

- 1 cup zucchini, chopped
- 2 cups low-sodium chicken broth
- 1/4 cup plain Greek yogurt

- 1 garlic clove, minced
- Salt and pepper to taste

Preparation:
1. In a pot, combine zucchini, chicken broth and garlic. Bring to a boil.
2. Reduce heat and simmer for 15 minutes until zucchini is tender.
3. Blend the mixture until smooth. Stir in Greek yogurt.
4. Season with salt and pepper before serving.

Comment: Light and creamy, this zucchini soup is both refreshing and satisfying. Perfect for gentle nourishment and easy digestion.

Nutritional info (per serving): Cal 70 | Carb 8g | Fat 2g | Prot 5g | Fib 1g.

22. BROCCOLI AND CHEESE SOUP

🔪 5 Min. ⏱ 15 Min. 🍽 2 Serv. 👨‍🍳 Easy

Ingredients:
- 1 cup broccoli florets
- 2 cups low-sodium vegetable broth
- 1/4 cup shredded cheddar cheese
- 1/4 cup plain Greek yogurt
- Salt and pepper to taste

Preparation:
1. In a pot, combine broccoli and vegetable broth. Bring to a boil.
2. Reduce heat and simmer for 10 minutes until broccoli is tender.
3. Use an immersion blender to puree the soup. Stir in the shredded cheese and Greek yogurt.
4. Season with salt and pepper to taste before serving.

Comment: The rich flavor of cheddar blends beautifully with tender broccoli for a creamy, hearty soup. A wholesome and comforting choice.

Nutritional info (per serving): Cal 120 | Carb 8g | Fat 6g | Prot 9g | Fib 2g.

23. Smooth Beet Soup

| ✎ 5 Min. | 🕐 20 Min. | 🍲 2 Serv. | ⚱ Easy |

Ingredients:

- 1 cup beets, peeled and chopped
- 2 cups low-sodium vegetable broth
- 1/4 cup coconut milk
- 1/4 tsp ginger, grated
- Salt to taste

Preparation:

1. In a pot, combine beets, vegetable broth and grated ginger. Bring to a boil.
2. Reduce heat and simmer for 15 minutes until beets are tender.
3. Use an immersion blender to puree the soup. Stir in coconut milk.
4. Season with salt before serving.

Comment: Vibrant in color and flavor, this beet soup is subtly sweet with a hint of ginger. A nutritious and light dish to brighten your day.

Nutritional info (per serving): Cal 90 | Carb 12g | Fat 4g | Prot 3g | Fib 3g.

24. Sweet Potato Coconut Soup

| ✎ 5 Min. | 🕐 20 Min. | 🍲 2 Serv. | ⚱ Easy |

Ingredients:

- 1 cup sweet potatoes, peeled and diced
- 2 cups low-sodium vegetable broth
- 1/4 cup coconut milk
- 1/4 tsp cinnamon
- Salt to taste

Preparation:

1. In a pot, combine sweet potatoes and vegetable broth. Bring to a boil.
2. Reduce heat and simmer for 15 minutes until sweet potatoes are tender.
3. Use an immersion blender to puree the soup. Stir in coconut milk and cinnamon.
4. Season with salt before serving.

Comment: The natural sweetness of sweet potatoes pairs perfectly with the creamy coconut milk. A warm and satisfying soup for light eating.

Nutritional info (per serving): Cal 130 | Carb 20g | Fat 5g | Prot 2g | Fib 4g.

25. Silken Tofu and Spinach Soup

🔪 5 Min. ⏱ 10 Min. 🍽 2 Serv. 👨‍🍳 Easy

Ingredients:
- 1 cup spinach leaves
- 1/2 cup silken tofu, cubed
- 2 cups low-sodium vegetable broth
- 1/4 tsp garlic powder
- Salt to taste

Preparation:
1. In a pot, bring the vegetable broth to a simmer. Add spinach and garlic powder.
2. Simmer for 5 minutes until spinach is wilted.
3. Add silken tofu and cook for an additional 2 minutes.
4. Season with salt before serving.

Comment: This protein-packed soup combines the smooth texture of tofu with the freshness of spinach. A simple and nourishing choice.

Nutritional info (per serving): Cal 70 | Carb 5g | Fat 3g | Prot 6g | Fib 1g.

26. Blended Oatmeal Smoothie

🔪 5 Min. ⏱ 0 Min. 🍽 2 Serv. 👨‍🍳 Easy

Ingredients:
- 1/2 cup rolled oats
- 1 cup unsweetened almond milk
- 1/4 cup Greek yogurt
- 1/2 banana
- 1 tsp honey (optional)

Preparation:
1. In a blender, combine oats, almond milk, Greek yogurt and banana.
2. Blend until smooth. Add honey for sweetness if desired.
3. Pour into glasses and serve chilled.

Comment: This creamy smoothie is a perfect blend of oats and banana, providing long-lasting energy and balanced nutrition.

Nutritional info (per serving): Cal 150 | Carb 24g | Fat 4g | Prot 5g | Fib 3g.

27. Berry Protein Shake

🥄 5 Min. ⏱ 0 Min. 🍽 2 Serv. 🗜 Easy

Ingredients:
- 1 cup mixed berries (frozen)
- 1 cup unsweetened almond milk
- 1 scoop unflavored protein powder
- 1/2 banana
- 1 tsp honey (optional)

Preparation:
1. In a blender, combine berries, almond milk, protein powder and banana.
2. Blend until smooth. Add honey if desired for sweetness.
3. Serve immediately.

Comment: Packed with berries and protein, this shake is both flavorful and nutritious. A refreshing boost to support your diet.

Nutritional info (per serving): Cal 130 | Carb 24g | Fat 2g | Prot 8g | Fib 3g.

28. Green Detox Shake

🥄 5 Min. ⏱ 0 Min. 🍽 2 Serv. 🗜 Easy

Ingredients:
- 1 cup spinach leaves
- 1/2 cucumber, peeled and chopped
- 1/2 green apple, cored and sliced
- 1 cup water
- 1 tsp lemon juice

Preparation:
1. In a blender, combine spinach, cucumber, apple, water and lemon juice.
2. Blend until smooth.
3. Serve chilled.

Comment: This vibrant shake combines spinach and cucumber for a hydrating, low-calorie drink. A great choice to recharge your day.

Nutritional info (per serving): Cal 50 | Carb 12g | Fat 0g | Prot 1g | Fib 2g.

29. Peanut Butter Banana Smoothie

🔪 5 Min. 🕐 0 Min. 🍽 2 Serv. 🍳 Easy

Ingredients:
- 1 banana
- 1 cup unsweetened almond milk
- 1 tbsp peanut butter
- 1/4 cup Greek yogurt
- 1 tsp honey (optional)

Preparation:
1. In a blender, combine banana, almond milk, peanut butter and Greek yogurt.
2. Blend until smooth. Add honey if desired for extra sweetness.
3. Serve chilled.

Comment: Creamy and rich, this smoothie combines the natural sweetness of banana with the indulgence of peanut butter. A filling and delicious treat.

Nutritional info (per serving): Cal 180 | Carb 24g | Fat 7g | Prot 6g | Fib 2g.

30. Creamy Chia Seed Shake

🔪 5+30 Min. 🕐 0 Min. 🍽 2 Serv. 🍳 Easy

Ingredients:
- 1 cup unsweetened almond milk
- 2 tbsp chia seeds
- 1/4 cup Greek yogurt
- 1/2 tsp vanilla extract
- 1 tsp honey

Preparation:
1. In a bowl, combine almond milk and chia seeds. Stir well and let soak for 30 minutes.
2. Transfer the mixture to a blender. Add Greek yogurt, vanilla extract and honey.

3. Blend until smooth. Serve chilled.

Comment: Chia seeds and almond milk make this shake creamy and nutrient-rich, while vanilla adds a hint of sweetness. Light and satisfying.

Nutritional info (per serving): Cal 100 | Carb 14g | Fat 4g | Prot 4g | Fib 3g.

31. Strawberry Kefir Smoothie

🔪 5 Min.　🕐 0 Min.　🍲 2 Serv.　🫙 Easy

Ingredients:
- 1 cup strawberries (fresh or frozen)
- 1 cup plain kefir
- 1/2 banana
- 1 tsp honey (optional)

Preparation:
1. In a blender, combine strawberries, kefir and banana.
2. Blend until smooth. Add honey if desired for sweetness.
3. Serve immediately.

Comment: A refreshing blend of strawberries and creamy kefir, this smoothie is naturally sweet and perfect for light nourishment.

Nutritional info (per serving): Cal 110 | Carb 19g | Fat 3g | Prot 4g | Fib 2g.

32. Tropical Mango Smoothie

🔪 5 Min.　🕐 0 Min.　🍲 2 Serv.　🫙 Easy

Ingredients:
- 1 cup mango chunks (fresh or frozen)
- 1 cup coconut water
- 1/2 cup Greek yogurt
- 1 tsp lime juice

Preparation:
1. In a blender, combine mango, coconut water, Greek yogurt and lime juice.
2. Blend until smooth.
3. Serve immediately.

Comment: The tropical sweetness of mango and the tang of Greek yogurt make this smoothie a delicious way to enjoy a sunny treat.

Nutritional info (per serving): Cal 120 | Carb 25g | Fat 1g | Prot 5g | Fib 2g.

33. Chocolate Avocado Shake

✎ 5 Min. ⏱ 0 Min. 🍲 2 Serv. 👨‍🍳 Easy

Ingredients:
- 1/2 avocado
- 1 cup unsweetened almond milk
- 1 tbsp cocoa powder
- 1 tbsp honey
- 1/2 tsp vanilla extract

Preparation:
1. In a blender, combine avocado, almond milk, cocoa powder, honey and vanilla extract.
2. Blend until smooth.
3. Serve chilled.

Comment: Smooth and rich, this chocolate shake is a guilt-free indulgence with the added creaminess of avocado.

Nutritional info (per serving): Cal 130 | Carb 16g | Fat 9g | Prot 3g | Fib 4g.

34. Apple Cinnamon Protein Shake

✎ 5 Min. ⏱ 0 Min. 🍲 2 Serv. 👨‍🍳 Easy

Ingredients:
- 1 cup unsweetened almond milk
- 1/2 apple, peeled and chopped
- 1/2 tsp cinnamon
- 1 scoop vanilla protein powder
- 1 tsp honey (optional)

Preparation:
1. In a blender, combine almond milk, apple, cinnamon and protein powder.
2. Blend until smooth. Add honey for sweetness if desired.

3. Serve chilled.

Comment: A warming combination of apple and cinnamon paired with protein for a filling, flavorful shake.

Nutritional info (per serving): Cal 120 | Carb 16g | Fat 2g | Prot 10g | Fib 3g.

35. Blueberry Almond Milk Smoothie

🔪 5 Min.   🕐 0 Min.   🍽 2 Serv.   ⚗ Easy

Ingredients:
- 1 cup blueberries (fresh or frozen)
- 1 cup unsweetened almond milk
- 1/4 cup Greek yogurt
- 1 tsp honey (optional)

Preparation:
1. In a blender, combine blueberries, almond milk and Greek yogurt.
2. Blend until smooth. Add honey if desired for sweetness.
3. Serve chilled.

Comment: Sweet blueberries blend perfectly with creamy almond milk and Greek yogurt for a balanced and refreshing drink.

Nutritional info (per serving): Cal 110 | Carb 18g | Fat 3g | Prot 4g | Fib 3g.

36. Iced Matcha Protein Shake

🔪 5 Min.   🕐 0 Min.   🍽 2 Serv.   ⚗ Easy

Ingredients:
- 1 cup unsweetened almond milk
- 1 tsp matcha powder
- 1 scoop vanilla protein powder
- 1/2 cup ice cubes
- 1 tsp honey (optional)

Preparation:
1. In a blender, combine almond milk, matcha powder, protein powder and ice cubes.
2. Blend until smooth and frothy. Add honey for sweetness if desired.

3. Serve immediately, chilled.

Comment: Energizing matcha combines with creamy almond milk and protein powder for a frothy, refreshing shake.

Nutritional info (per serving): Cal 100 | Carb 8g | Fat 3g | Prot 12g | Fib 1g.

37. Vanilla Chai Smoothie

🔪 5 Min. ⏱ 0 Min. 🍲 2 Serv. 👨‍🍳 Easy

Ingredients:
- 1 cup unsweetened almond milk
- 1/2 cup Greek yogurt
- 1/2 tsp chai spice blend
- 1/2 tsp vanilla extract
- 1 tsp honey (optional)

Preparation:
1. In a blender, combine almond milk, Greek yogurt, chai spice blend and vanilla extract.
2. Blend until smooth. Add honey if you prefer extra sweetness.
3. Serve chilled.

Comment: A cozy blend of chai spices and vanilla in a creamy smoothie that feels indulgent while staying light.

Nutritional info (per serving): Cal 90 | Carb 10g | Fat 3g | Prot 7g | Fib 2g.

38. Cucumber Mint Cooler

🔪 5 Min. ⏱ 0 Min. 🍲 2 Serv. 👨‍🍳 Easy

Ingredients:
- 1 cup cucumber, peeled and chopped
- 1/4 cup fresh mint leaves
- 1 cup water
- 1 tsp lemon juice
- 1 tsp honey (optional)

Preparation:
1. In a blender, combine cucumber, mint leaves, water and lemon juice.

2. Blend until smooth. Add honey for extra sweetness if desired.
3. Serve immediately, chilled.

Comment: Crisp cucumber and fresh mint create a hydrating drink that is both light and invigorating.

Nutritional info (per serving): Cal 20 | Carb 5g | Fat 0g | Prot 1g | Fib 1g.

39. WATERMELON COCONUT DRINK

> ✎ 5 Min. ⏱ 0 Min. 🍲 2 Serv. 👨‍🍳 Easy

Ingredients:
- 1 cup watermelon, cubed and seeds removed
- 1/2 cup coconut water
- 1/4 cup Greek yogurt
- 1 tsp lime juice

Preparation:
1. In a blender, combine watermelon, coconut water, Greek yogurt and lime juice.
2. Blend until smooth.
3. Serve immediately, chilled.

Comment: Sweet watermelon and creamy coconut water combine for a refreshing, tropical inspired drink.

Nutritional info (per serving): Cal 50 | Carb 11g | Fat 1g | Prot 2g | Fib 1g.

40. GOLDEN TURMERIC MILK

> ✎ 5 Min. ⏱ 5 Min. 🍲 2 Serv. 👨‍🍳 Easy

Ingredients:
- 1 cup unsweetened almond milk
- 1/2 tsp turmeric powder
- 1/4 tsp cinnamon
- 1/2 tsp honey (optional)
- 1/4 tsp vanilla extract

Preparation:
1. In a small saucepan, combine almond milk, turmeric powder, cinnamon and vanilla extract

2. Warm over medium heat for 3-5 minutes, stirring occasionally. Do not let it boil.
3. Remove from heat. Stir in honey if desired for sweetness.
4. Serve warm.

Comment: Warm and soothing, this turmeric milk offers subtle spices and creamy almond milk for a comforting, nutrient-rich beverage.

Nutritional info (per serving): Cal 40 | Carb 6g | Fat 2g | Prot 1g | Fib 1g.

Chapter 3: Phase 2 - Semisolid Diet

— ❖ —

Entering the semisolid diet phase is an exciting step forward. After weeks of liquids, your body is ready for foods with more texture and substance. This phase is all about exploring new, softer foods that are easy to digest while continuing to support your body's healing process. It's a gradual reintroduction, where you learn to listen closely to your body's cues and take time with each bite. With a focus on smooth, moist and nutrient-rich foods, this phase helps you rebuild a balanced eating routine that aligns with your new lifestyle.

Transition and suggestions

Moving into the semisolid diet phase is an exciting milestone on your journey. After weeks of relying solely on liquids, this stage allows you to start introducing a bit more texture and substance into your meals. Your stomach has had time to heal and adapt and now it's ready for the next step. However, this phase requires careful attention to ensure a smooth transition. Your digestive system is still adjusting, so the foods you choose need to be soft, easily chewable and gentle on the stomach.

The semisolid phase is about reintroducing food slowly, with a focus on nutrition and digestibility. You'll start to explore foods that have a bit more body than liquids but are still light enough to pass through your new, smaller stomach without causing discomfort. This is when you begin to retrain your palate and habits, learning what works for your body. It's a process of trial and error, where paying close attention to how different foods make you feel is key. Some foods might sit well, while others may not be as compatible and that's perfectly normal. This phase gives you the opportunity to experiment and find the balance that suits your unique needs.

Start with small portions, about the size of a golf ball or two tablespoons and eat slowly. It might be tempting to take bigger bites or eat more quickly, especially now that you're introducing new textures, but remember that your stomach can only handle so much at a time. Chewing thoroughly is crucial at this stage. Aim to chew each bite until it reaches a smooth, almost paste-like consistency. This not only aids in digestion but also helps prevent any feelings of discomfort or nausea that can come from swallowing larger pieces. Eating slowly allows you to tune in to your body's signals recognizing when you've had enough to feel satisfied.

When it comes to food choices, think soft, moist and easy to mash. Items like scrambled eggs, cottage cheese, yogurt, mashed vegetables and pureed fruits are excellent options to start with. Eggs, in particular, are a versatile and nutrient-dense choice. Softly scrambled or blended into a smooth consistency, they provide a good source of protein while being easy on the stomach. Cottage cheese and yogurt offer a creamy texture with added protein and probiotics, which support gut health. Choose plain, unsweetened varieties and consider adding a small amount of pureed fruit or a sprinkle of cinnamon to enhance flavor without adding unnecessary sugars.

Mashed vegetables, like sweet potatoes, carrots or cauliflower, introduce valuable vitamins and minerals into your diet while still being gentle on your digestive system. Steaming vegetables until they're very soft and mashing them with a bit of broth or milk creates a smooth, easily consumable dish. Similarly, pureed fruits like apples, pears or peaches offer a natural sweetness and provide fiber that aids in digestion. If needed, you can add a touch of cinnamon or nutmeg to give them more depth of flavor.

As you progress through this phase, you might find that certain proteins, like tender chicken or fish, can be blended or mashed into a more semisolid form. Shredded chicken mixed with a bit of broth or mashed avocado can be a filling and nutritious option. The key is to introduce these foods in small amounts and monitor how your stomach reacts. Protein continues to be a top priority, so including these softer protein sources helps you meet your daily needs without overwhelming your digestive system.

Hydration remains vital during the semisolid phase, but the way you approach drinking should be the same as in the liquid phase. Keep sipping fluids throughout the day, but avoid drinking during meals. It's easy to slip back into old habits, especially as foods start to resemble what you may have been used to before surgery. However, drinking while eating can still cause discomfort and can interfere with the signals of fullness your stomach is trying to send. Waiting at least 30 minutes after a meal before drinking fluids helps maintain that feeling of satisfaction and allows food to digest properly.

As you explore different foods, it's also important to keep track of any patterns. If you notice certain foods cause discomfort, bloating or an upset stomach, make a note and consider trying them again at a later time. Your stomach is still healing and foods that may not agree with you now could become tolerable in the future. The semisolid phase is a learning process, teaching you how to navigate your new dietary landscape with flexibility and patience.

Another useful tip during this phase is to focus on foods that combine nutrition with ease of preparation. Smooth soups made with blended vegetables and a protein base, such as pureed lentil or split pea soup, can offer a satisfying, nutrient-rich option. Similarly, low-fat refried beans with a bit of melted cheese can provide both protein and a creamy texture that is easy to consume. The idea is to keep meals simple yet nourishing, avoiding overly processed foods or those with added sugars and unhealthy fats.

Embracing the semisolid phase means embracing the idea of mindful eating. Meals are no longer just about filling up; they're about providing your body with what it truly needs to thrive. This phase is a balance between introducing variety and respecting the limits of your stomach. As you experiment with different foods and flavors, remember that there's no rush. Take each meal as an opportunity to nurture your body and build a positive relationship with eating. By the end of this phase, you'll have gained a clearer understanding of what foods work best for you, laying the foundation for the next step in your post-surgery journey.

Semisolid Recipes

❖

41. Creamy Mashed Cauliflower

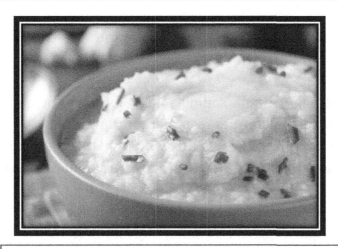

🔪 5 Min.　🕐 15 Min.　🍲 2 Serv.　🧂 Easy

Ingredients:

- 2 cups cauliflower florets
- 1/4 cup plain Greek yogurt
- 1 tbsp grated Parmesan cheese
- 1 clove garlic, minced
- Salt and pepper to taste

Preparation:

1. Steam cauliflower florets for about 10 minutes until tender.
2. Transfer the cauliflower to a bowl and add Greek yogurt, Parmesan cheese and minced garlic.
3. Use a fork or an immersion blender to mash until smooth.
4. Season with salt and pepper to taste before serving.

Comment: This creamy mashed cauliflower offers a delightful alternative to traditional mashed potatoes, with a smooth texture and a subtle garlic-Parmesan flavor.

Nutritional info (per serving): Cal 80 | Carb 10g | Fat 3g | Prot 5g | Fib 3g.

42. Soft Scrambled Eggs with Cheese

📝 5 Min.   🕐 5 Min.   🍽 2 Serv.   👨‍🍳 Easy

Ingredients:
- 2 large eggs
- 1/4 cup shredded cheddar cheese
- 2 tbsp milk
- 1/2 tbsp butter
- Salt and pepper to taste

Preparation:
1. In a bowl, whisk eggs with milk and a pinch of salt and pepper.
2. In a nonstick skillet, melt butter over medium-low heat.
3. Pour in the egg mixture and stir gently with a spatula until curds form.
4. Add the shredded cheese and stir until eggs are soft and creamy. Serve immediately.

Comment: Soft and creamy, these scrambled eggs combine the richness of cheddar with the fluffiness of perfectly cooked eggs for a comforting and protein-rich meal.

Nutritional info (per serving): Cal 140 | Carb 1g | Fat 11g | Prot 10g | Fib 0g.

43. Smooth Cottage Cheese and Avocado Mix

📝 5 Min.   🕐 0 Min.   🍽 2 Serv.   👨‍🍳 Easy

Ingredients:
- 1/2 cup cottage cheese
- 1/2 avocado, peeled and pitted
- 1 tsp lemon juice
- Salt and pepper to taste
- 1 tbsp fresh chives, chopped (optional)

Preparation:
1. In a bowl, mash the avocado until smooth.
2. Add cottage cheese and lemon juice to the avocado, mixing until well combined.
3. Season with salt and pepper to taste. Sprinkle with chopped chives if desired.

Comment: The creaminess of cottage cheese paired with the richness of avocado creates a simple yet luxurious blend, perfect for light and nutritious eating.

Nutritional info (per serving): Cal 90 | Carb 4g | Fat 6g | Prot 6g | Fib 2g.

44. MASHED SWEET POTATO DELIGHT

🔪 10 Min. 🕐 15 Min. 🍲 2 Serv. 👨‍🍳 Easy

Ingredients:
- 1 cup sweet potato, peeled and diced
- 1/4 cup plain Greek yogurt
- 1/4 tsp cinnamon
- Salt to taste
- 1 tsp honey (optional)

Preparation:
1. Boil sweet potato pieces for 10 minutes or until tender. Drain and transfer to a bowl.
2. Add Greek yogurt and cinnamon to the sweet potatoes. Mash until smooth.
3. Season with salt and stir in honey if desired. Serve warm.

Comment: Sweet potato mash gets a flavorful twist with Greek yogurt and cinnamon, creating a warm, naturally sweet dish that's light yet satisfying.

Nutritional info (per serving): Cal 110 | Carb 24g | Fat 1g | Prot 3g | Fib 4g.

45. SILKY PUMPKIN PUREE

🔪 5 Min. 🕐 10 Min. 🍲 2 Serv. 👨‍🍳 Easy

Ingredients:
- 1 cup canned pumpkin puree
- 1/4 cup coconut milk
- 1/4 tsp nutmeg
- 1/4 tsp cinnamon
- Salt to taste

Preparation:
1. In a small saucepan, combine pumpkin puree, coconut milk, nutmeg and cinnamon.
2. Warm over medium heat for 5-7 minutes, stirring occasionally.
3. Season with salt to taste and serve warm.

Comment: This silky pumpkin puree blends warm spices with the creaminess of coconut milk, delivering a comforting and nutrient-rich dish in every spoonful.

Nutritional info (per serving): Cal 80 | Carb 12g | Fat 4g | Prot 2g | Fib 3g.

46. Creamy Spinach and Ricotta Blend

✎ 5 Min. ⏱ 5 Min. 🍲 2 Serv. 🍶 Easy

Ingredients:
- 1 cup fresh spinach leaves
- 1/4 cup ricotta cheese
- 1 tbsp plain Greek yogurt
- 1 garlic clove, minced
- Salt and pepper to taste

Preparation:
1. In a skillet, sauté spinach and garlic over medium heat until wilted (about 2 minutes).
2. Transfer the spinach to a bowl. Add ricotta cheese and Greek yogurt.
3. Mix until smooth and creamy. Season with salt and pepper to taste.

Comment: A combination of sautéed spinach and creamy ricotta, this dish is rich in flavor yet light enough for a balanced meal or side dish.

Nutritional info (per serving): Cal 90 | Carb 5g | Fat 5g | Prot 6g | Fib 2g.

47. Soft Tofu and Berry Parfait

✎ 5 Min. ⏱ 0 Min. 🍲 2 Serv. 🍶 Easy

Ingredients:
- 1/2 cup silken tofu
- 1/2 cup mixed berries
- 1 tsp honey
- 1/4 tsp vanilla extract
- 1 tbsp chia seeds (optional)

Preparation:
1. In a blender, combine silken tofu, honey and vanilla extract. Blend until smooth.
2. In small serving cups, layer the tofu mixture with mixed berries.
3. Sprinkle with chia seeds if desired. Serve immediately or chilled.

Comment: This parfait layers silky tofu with sweet mixed berries for a refreshing and protein-packed dessert that's light and easy to enjoy.

Nutritional info (per serving): Cal 100 | Carb 16g | Fat 3g | Prot 5g | Fib 3g.

48. Savory Ricotta and Herb Mash

✎ 5 Min. ⏲ 5 Min. ◎ 2 Serv. ♨ Easy

Ingredients:
- 1/2 cup ricotta cheese
- 1/4 cup steamed broccoli florets
- 1 tbsp fresh basil, chopped
- 1 garlic clove, minced
- Salt and pepper to taste

Preparation:
1. In a bowl, combine ricotta cheese, steamed broccoli, basil and minced garlic.
2. Use a fork to mash the ingredients until smooth.
3. Season with salt and pepper to taste. Serve warm.

Comment: A creamy ricotta mash enriched with fresh herbs and tender broccoli creates a savory and versatile dish that's simple yet flavorful.

Nutritional info (per serving): Cal 90 | Carb 4g | Fat 5g | Prot 6g | Fib 2g.

49. Creamy Butternut Squash and Carrot Blend

✎ 10 Min. ⏲ 15 Min. ◎ 2 Serv. ♨ Easy

Ingredients:
- 1 cup butternut squash, peeled and diced
- 1/2 cup carrots, peeled and diced
- 1/4 cup coconut milk
- 1/4 tsp ground ginger
- Salt to taste

Preparation:
1. Boil squash and carrot pieces for 10 minutes or until tender. Drain and transfer to a bowl.
2. Add coconut milk and ground ginger. Mash until smooth.
3. Season with salt to taste and serve warm.

Comment: Butternut squash and carrots come together in this creamy blend, with coconut milk and ginger adding a hint of sweetness and warmth.

Nutritional info (per serving): Cal 100 | Carb 16g | Fat 4g | Prot 2g | Fib 3g.

50. Blended Chickpea and Tahini Puree

🔪 5 Min.   🕐 5 Min.   🍽 2 Serv.   🍳 Easy

Ingredients:
- 1/2 cup canned chickpeas, rinsed and drained
- 1 tbsp tahini
- 1 tbsp lemon juice
- 1 garlic clove, minced
- Salt to taste

Preparation:
1. In a blender, combine chickpeas, tahini, lemon juice and minced garlic.
2. Blend until smooth. If the mixture is too thick, add a splash of water.
3. Season with salt to taste and serve.

Comment: Chickpeas and tahini create a smooth and flavorful puree, enhanced by lemon and garlic for a light yet protein-rich dish.

Nutritional info (per serving): Cal 120 | Carb 14g | Fat 6g | Prot 5g | Fib 4g.

51. Creamy Lentil Mash with Herbs

🔪 10 Min.   🕐 15 Min.   🍽 2 Serv.   🍳 Easy

Ingredients:
- 1/2 cup red lentils
- 1 cup water
- 1 tbsp plain Greek yogurt
- 1 tsp fresh parsley, chopped
- Salt and pepper to taste

Preparation:
1. In a pot, combine lentils and water. Bring to a boil, then simmer for 10-12 minutes until tender.

2. Drain any excess water. Transfer lentils to a bowl and add Greek yogurt.
3. Mash until smooth. Stir in chopped parsley and season with salt and pepper.

Comment: This lentil mash is packed with plant-based protein and a creamy texture, enhanced by the fresh, vibrant touch of parsley for a wholesome and satisfying dish.

Nutritional info (per serving): Cal 90 | Carb 16g | Fat 1g | Prot 6g | Fib 3g.

52. Smooth Apple-Cinnamon Oatmeal

🔪 5 Min. 🕐 5 Min. 🍽 2 Serv. 👨‍🍳 Easy

Ingredients:
- 1/2 cup quick oats
- 1 cup water
- 1/2 apple, peeled and finely grated
- 1/4 tsp cinnamon
- 1 tsp honey (optional)

Preparation:
1. In a saucepan, combine oats and water. Cook over medium heat for 3-4 minutes, stirring occasionally.
2. Add grated apple and cinnamon. Stir well and cook for another minute.
3. Drizzle with honey if desired. Serve warm.

Comment: Combining the natural sweetness of apples with the warmth of cinnamon, this oatmeal is a cozy and nutritious breakfast option that's ready in minutes.

Nutritional info (per serving): Cal 90 | Carb 19g | Fat 1g | Prot 3g | Fib 3g.

53. Greek Yogurt and Honey Swirl

🔪 5 Min. 🕐 0 Min. 🍽 2 Serv. 👨‍🍳 Easy

Ingredients:
- 1 cup Greek yogurt
- 1 tbsp honey
- 1/4 tsp vanilla extract
- 1 tbsp chopped nuts (optional)

Preparation:

1. In a bowl, combine Greek yogurt and vanilla extract.
2. Swirl in the honey using a spoon.
3. Top with chopped nuts if desired. Serve immediately.

Comment: The simplicity of Greek yogurt is elevated with a swirl of honey and a hint of vanilla, creating a creamy, protein-rich snack or light dessert.

Nutritional info (per serving): Cal 110 | Carb 14g | Fat 3g | Prot 8g | Fib 0g.

54. Mango Chia Seed Pudding

🔪 5+30 Min. ⏱ 0 Min. 🍽 2 Serv. 👨‍🍳 Easy

Ingredients:
- 1/2 cup coconut milk
- 1 tbsp chia seeds
- 1/2 cup mango, pureed
- 1/4 tsp vanilla extract
- 1 tsp honey (optional)

Preparation:
1. In a bowl, combine coconut milk, chia seeds and vanilla extract. Stir well.
2. Let the mixture sit for 30 minutes until it thickens.
3. Layer the chia pudding with mango puree in serving cups. Add honey for extra sweetness if desired.

Comment: This pudding combines the tropical sweetness of mango with the creamy texture of chia seeds, offering a nutrient-packed and refreshing treat.

Nutritional info (per serving): Cal 120 | Carb 16g | Fat 6g | Prot 2g | Fib 4g.

55. Silky Carrot and Ginger Mash

🔪 10 Min. ⏱ 15 Min. 🍽 2 Serv. 👨‍🍳 Easy

Ingredients:
- 1 cup carrots, peeled and chopped
- 1/4 cup coconut milk
- 1/4 tsp grated ginger
- Salt to taste
- 1 tsp honey (optional)

Preparation:
1. Boil carrot pieces for 10 minutes or until tender. Drain and transfer to a bowl.
2. Add coconut milk and grated ginger. Mash until smooth.
3. Season with salt and stir in honey if desired. Serve warm.

Comment: The natural sweetness of carrots pairs beautifully with the warmth of ginger and the richness of coconut milk, resulting in a velvety and aromatic mash.

Nutritional info (per serving): Cal 80 | Carb 11g | Fat 4g | Prot 2g | Fib 3g.

56. Mashed Avocado with Soft-Boiled Egg

✎ 5 Min. ◷ 5 Min. ◎ 2 Serv. ⚗ Easy

Ingredients:
- 1 ripe avocado, peeled and pitted
- 2 large eggs
- 1 tsp lemon juice
- Salt and pepper to taste
- 1 tbsp fresh parsley, chopped (optional)

Preparation:
1. Bring a pot of water to a boil. Gently place the eggs in and cook for 4 minutes for a soft-boiled consistency.
2. While the eggs cook, mash the avocado in a bowl and mix in the lemon juice. Season with salt and pepper.
3. Peel the eggs, chop them and gently mix into the mashed avocado.
4. Garnish with parsley if desired. Serve immediately.

Comment: Creamy mashed avocado meets the delicate texture of soft-boiled eggs in this simple yet satisfying dish, perfect for a nutrient-dense meal or snack.

Nutritional info (per serving): Cal 170 | Carb 6g | Fat 14g | Prot 8g | Fib 5g.

57. Soft Banana and Greek Yogurt Blend

✎ 5 Min.   🕐 0 Min.   🍳 2 Serv.   ♟ Easy

Ingredients:
- 1 ripe banana
- 1/2 cup Greek yogurt
- 1/4 tsp cinnamon
- 1 tsp honey (optional)
- 1 tbsp chia seeds (optional)

Preparation:
1. In a bowl, mash the banana until smooth.
2. Mix in the Greek yogurt and cinnamon until well combined.
3. Add honey for extra sweetness if desired. Sprinkle with chia seeds for added texture.

Comment: This creamy blend of ripe banana and Greek yogurt, with a hint of cinnamon, is a light yet energizing option for a quick breakfast or snack.

Nutritional info (per serving): Cal 120 | Carb 21g | Fat 2g | Prot 5g | Fib 2g.

58. Ricotta and Spinach Puree

✎ 5 Min.   🕐 5 Min.   🍳 2 Serv.   ♟ Easy

Ingredients:
- 1 cup fresh spinach leaves
- 1/2 cup ricotta cheese
- 1 clove garlic, minced
- 1/4 tsp nutmeg
- Salt and pepper to taste

Preparation:
1. In a skillet, sauté spinach and garlic over medium heat for 2 minutes until wilted.
2. Transfer to a blender, add ricotta cheese and nutmeg and blend until smooth.
3. Season with salt and pepper to taste. Serve warm.

Comment: Sautéed spinach and creamy ricotta come together in this savory puree, enhanced by a hint of nutmeg for a flavorful and balanced dish.

Nutritional info (per serving): Cal 100 | Carb 4g | Fat 5g | Prot 7g | Fib 2g.

59. Soft Pea and Mint Mash

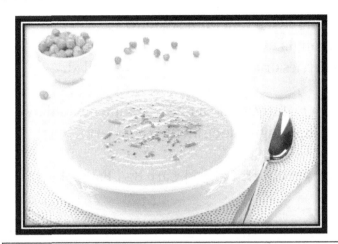

🔪 5 Min. 🕐 10 Min. 🍽 2 Serv. 👨‍🍳 Easy

Ingredients:
- 1 cup frozen peas
- 1/4 cup Greek yogurt
- 1 tbsp fresh mint leaves, chopped
- 1 tsp lemon juice
- Salt to taste

Preparation:
1. Boil peas for 5 minutes until tender. Drain and transfer to a bowl.
2. Add Greek yogurt, mint and lemon juice to the peas. Mash until smooth.
3. Season with salt to taste and serve warm.

Comment: This pea and mint mash is refreshing and creamy, with a zesty hint of lemon and a smooth texture that makes it a delightful addition to any meal.

Nutritional info (per serving): Cal 80 | Carb 14g | Fat 1g | Prot 5g | Fib 4g.

60. Silken Tofu with Honey and Vanilla

🔪 5 Min. 🕐 0 Min. 🍽 2 Serv. 👨‍🍳 Easy

Ingredients:
- 1/2 cup silken tofu
- 1 tsp honey
- 1/4 tsp vanilla extract

- 1 tbsp fresh berries (optional)
- 1 tbsp chopped nuts (optional)

Preparation:
1. In a bowl, mash the silken tofu until smooth.
2. Add honey and vanilla extract, mixing well.
3. Top with fresh berries or nuts if desired. Serve chilled.

Comment: The smooth texture of silken tofu is complemented by a drizzle of honey and a touch of vanilla, making this a simple, light, and satisfying dessert.

Nutritional info (per serving): Cal 70 | Carb 8g | Fat 3g | Prot 4g | Fib 1g.

61. Smooth Sweet Potato and Cinnamon Mix

✎ 5 Min.   🕐 15 Min.   🍽 2 Serv.   👨‍🍳 Easy

Ingredients:
- 1 cup sweet potato, peeled and diced
- 1/4 cup plain Greek yogurt
- 1/2 tsp cinnamon
- 1 tsp honey (optional)
- Salt to taste

Preparation:
1. Boil sweet potato pieces for 10 minutes or until tender. Drain and transfer to a bowl.
2. Add Greek yogurt and cinnamon. Mash until smooth.
3. Add honey if desired and season with salt to taste. Serve warm.

Comment: The natural sweetness of the sweet potato combines beautifully with the warm spice of cinnamon, creating a creamy and comforting dish that's perfect for any time of the day.

Nutritional info (per serving): Cal 110 | Carb 24g | Fat 1g | Prot 3g | Fib 4g.

62. Blended Chicken and Broccoli Mash

✎ 10 Min.   🕐 15 Min.   🍽 2 Serv.   👨‍🍳 Easy

Ingredients:
- 1/2 cup cooked chicken breast, shredded
- 1 cup broccoli florets

- 1/4 cup plain Greek yogurt
- 1/4 tsp garlic powder
- Salt and pepper to taste

Preparation:
1. Steam broccoli for 5 minutes until tender.
2. In a blender, combine cooked chicken, broccoli, Greek yogurt and garlic powder. Blend until smooth.
3. Season with salt and pepper to taste. Serve warm.

Comment: This high-protein blend of tender chicken and broccoli delivers a creamy texture and a rich flavor, making it both nourishing and satisfying.

Nutritional info (per serving): Cal 130 | Carb 6g | Fat 3g | Prot 20g | Fib 2g.

63. CREAMY POLENTA WITH PARMESAN

✎ 5 Min. ⏱ 10 Min. 📷 2 Serv. 🍴 Easy

Ingredients:
- 1/4 cup polenta (cornmeal)
- 1 cup water
- 1/4 cup grated Parmesan cheese
- 1 tbsp Greek yogurt
- Salt to taste

Preparation:
1. In a pot, bring water to a boil. Gradually add polenta, stirring continuously.
2. Reduce heat and cook for 5-7 minutes, stirring until thickened.
3. Remove from heat and stir in Parmesan cheese and Greek yogurt.
4. Season with salt to taste. Serve warm.

Comment: Smooth and creamy, this Parmesan-infused polenta offers a savory, melt-in-your-mouth experience with a light and satisfying finish.

Nutritional info (per serving): Cal 120 | Carb 16g | Fat 4g | Prot 6g | Fib 1g.

64. Mashed Cauliflower and Cheddar Blend

🔪 10 Min. 🕐 15 Min. 🍽 2 Serv. 👨‍🍳 Easy

Ingredients:

- 2 cups cauliflower florets
- 1/4 cup shredded cheddar cheese
- 1 tbsp plain Greek yogurt
- Salt and pepper to taste
- 1 clove garlic, minced (optional)

Preparation:

1. Steam cauliflower florets for about 10 minutes until tender.
2. Transfer the cauliflower to a bowl, add cheese, Greek yogurt and minced garlic if using.
3. Mash until smooth. Season with salt and pepper to taste.

Comment: The subtle flavor of cauliflower blends perfectly with sharp cheddar cheese, creating a creamy mash that's rich in taste yet light on calories.

Nutritional info (per serving): Cal 100 | Carb 8g | Fat 6g | Prot 6g | Fib 3g.

65. Soft Baked Apple and Cinnamon Mix

🔪 5 Min. 🕐 15 Min. 🍽 2 Serv. 👨‍🍳 Easy

Ingredients:

- 1 apple, peeled, cored and sliced
- 1/4 cup water
- 1/2 tsp cinnamon
- 1 tsp honey (optional)
- 1 tbsp Greek yogurt

Preparation:

1. In a small saucepan, combine apple slices, water and cinnamon. Cook over medium heat for 10 minutes until apples are soft.
2. Mash the apples with a fork. Stir in honey if desired and Greek yogurt.
3. Serve warm.

Comment: Soft baked apples with a touch of cinnamon deliver a naturally sweet and warming dish enhanced by the creaminess of Greek yogurt for a perfect balance.

Nutritional info (per serving): Cal 70 | Carb 18g | Fat 0g | Prot 1g | Fib 3g.

66. Creamy Pumpkin and Quinoa Mash

✎ 10 Min. ⏱ 15 Min. 🍽 2 Serv. 👨‍🍳 Easy

Ingredients:
- 1/4 cup quinoa
- 1 cup water
- 1/2 cup canned pumpkin puree
- 1/4 tsp nutmeg
- Salt to taste

Preparation:
1. In a pot, bring water to a boil. Add quinoa, reduce heat and simmer for 10 minutes.
2. Drain excess water and mix quinoa with pumpkin puree and nutmeg.
3. Season with salt to taste and serve warm.

Comment: Nutty quinoa meets creamy pumpkin in this satisfying dish, with a hint of nutmeg adding warmth and depth to the flavor.

Nutritional info (per serving): Cal 100 | Carb 18g | Fat 2g | Prot 3g | Fib 2g.

67. Mashed Black Beans and Avocado

✎ 5 Min. ⏱ 5 Min. 🍽 2 Serv. 👨‍🍳 Easy

Ingredients:
- 1/2 cup canned black beans, rinsed and drained
- 1/2 avocado, peeled and pitted
- 1 tsp lime juice
- Salt and pepper to taste
- 1 tbsp chopped cilantro (optional)

Preparation:
1. In a bowl, mash the black beans and avocado together until smooth.
2. Add lime juice and mix well. Season with salt and pepper to taste.
3. Garnish with cilantro if desired.

Comment: This creamy mash of black beans and avocado, with a hint of lime and optional cilantro, is both nutritious and bursting with vibrant flavor.

Nutritional info (per serving): Cal 110 | Carb 13g | Fat 6g | Prot 3g | Fib 5g.

68. Smooth Zucchini and Potato Blend

✎ 10 Min.   ⏱ 15 Min.   🍲 2 Serv.   ♟ Easy

Ingredients:
- 1 cup zucchini, chopped
- 1 small potato, peeled and chopped
- 1/4 cup plain Greek yogurt
- Salt and pepper to taste
- 1/2 tsp garlic powder (optional)

Preparation:
1. Boil zucchini and potato for 10 minutes or until tender. Drain and transfer to a bowl.
2. Add Greek yogurt and garlic powder if using. Mash until smooth.
3. Season with salt and pepper to taste. Serve warm.

Comment: The delicate flavors of zucchini and potato are combined into a creamy and smooth mash, made even more delightful with a touch of Greek yogurt.

Nutritional info (per serving): Cal 80 | Carb 17g | Fat 1g | Prot 3g | Fib 2g.

69. Soft Cottage Cheese with Peaches

✎ 5 Min.   ⏱ 0 Min.   🍲 2 Serv.   ♟ Easy

Ingredients:
- 1/2 cup cottage cheese
- 1/2 cup peaches, peeled and diced
- 1 tsp honey
- 1/4 tsp cinnamon
- 1 tbsp chopped nuts (optional)

Preparation:
1. In a bowl, combine cottage cheese, diced peaches, honey and cinnamon.
2. Mix until well combined. Top with chopped nuts if desired.
3. Serve chilled.

Comment: Fresh peaches paired with creamy cottage cheese create a naturally sweet and light dish, with a hint of cinnamon adding warmth and depth.

Nutritional info (per serving): Cal 90 | Carb 14g | Fat 2g | Prot 5g | Fib 1g.

70. Creamy Rice Pudding with Nutmeg

✎ 5 Min. ⏱ 15 Min. 🍽 2 Serv. 🍳 Easy

Ingredients:
- 1/4 cup cooked rice
- 1/2 cup milk
- 1 tbsp honey
- 1/4 tsp nutmeg
- 1/4 tsp vanilla extract

Preparation:
1. In a small saucepan, combine cooked rice, milk, honey and nutmeg.
2. Cook over medium heat for 5-7 minutes until thickened, stirring frequently.
3. Stir in vanilla extract and serve warm.

Comment: This creamy rice pudding, subtly spiced with nutmeg and sweetened with honey, delivers a rich and comforting dessert or snack.

Nutritional info (per serving): Cal 110 | Carb 20g | Fat 2g | Prot 3g | Fib 1g.

Chapter 4: Phase 3 - Solid Diet

---------- ❖ ----------

Entering the solid diet phase is a significant achievement, marking a new level of normalcy in your eating habits. Your body has gradually adapted and now it's ready to handle more complex textures and a wider variety of foods. This phase is about reintroducing solid foods with care, ensuring that each meal is balanced, nutritious and easy for your stomach to manage. It's a time to experiment with different flavors, savor each bite and continue building the mindful eating habits you've developed. Your focus remains on choosing quality over quantity, letting your body guide you toward what feels best.

Reinsert solid foods gradually

Transitioning to solid foods is a major milestone in your journey. It signifies that your body has healed enough to handle more complex textures and a wider variety of nutrients. However, this phase is not about diving headfirst into your pre-surgery eating habits. It requires a thoughtful, gradual approach, reintroducing solids one step at a time to ensure that your stomach adapts smoothly. Your digestive system is still learning how to process food in its new form, so easing into this phase will help you identify what works best for you and what might still be challenging.

The focus now shifts to small, nutrient-dense meals that you can chew thoroughly and digest comfortably. It's important to start with foods that are tender, moist and easy to break down in your mouth. Think of soft-cooked vegetables, flaky fish, ground meats and tender poultry. These choices are not only easier to chew, but they're also less likely to cause discomfort as they pass through your smaller stomach. Introducing solid foods gradually gives your digestive system the time it needs to acclimate to the increased complexity of textures. This period is about finding balance, learning to savor each bite and recognizing when your body signals that it's had enough.

Chewing is more crucial now than ever. When you reintroduce solid foods, aim to chew each bite until it reaches an almost paste-like consistency. This habit helps reduce the workload on your stomach, making digestion easier and minimizing the risk of any blockages or discomfort. It also encourages mindful eating, giving you the time to fully experience the flavors and textures of each meal. Rushing through meals or swallowing chunks of food can lead to unpleasant sensations, so slowing down becomes an essential practice. It might feel tedious at first, but this careful approach will become second nature as you settle into this phase.

Portion sizes continue to be small, usually around half a cup to a cup per meal, depending on how your body responds. Your stomach's capacity remains limited, so it's about quality over quantity. Choose foods that are rich in protein, vitamins and minerals, as these will provide the most benefi in small amounts. Proteins like shredded chicken, turkey or soft, flaky fish are great starting points. They offer the nutrients your body needs for muscle maintenance and energy, while their texture makes them easier to chew and digest. If meat feels too heavy initially, consider incorporating soft plant-based proteins like tofu or well-cooked legumes into your meals.

Vegetables now make a more prominent appearance, but they should be cooked until they're soft and tender. Raw, crunchy vegetables might be too harsh on your digestive system at this stage, so steaming, roasting or sautéing them in a bit of broth or olive oil is the way to go. Carrots, zucchini, spinach and squash are excellent options to start with. Their natural flavors, paired with simple seasonings, can create satisfying and nutritious sides that complement your protein sources. As with everything, introduce them one at a time and monitor how your body reacts. This careful experimentation helps you build a list of foods that work well with your new dietary needs.

Fruits can also be reintroduced gradually, focusing on softer varieties like bananas, ripe pears or applesauce. Avoid fruits with tough skins or high acidity until you're confident your stomach can handle them. Peeling and mashing fruits can make them easier to digest and allow you to enjoy their natural sweetness without overwhelming your system. As you become more comfortable, you can slowly expand to other types of fruits, always paying attention to how your body responds.

This phase also marks the reintroduction of complex carbohydrates, though in moderation. Soft grains like quinoa, oatmeal and well-cooked rice can be added to your meals in small quantities. They provide fiber and energy, supporting digestion and helping you feel more satisfied. However, it's important to keep portions controlled and to pair them with protein and vegetables to create a balanced meal. Heavy or refined carbs, like bread, pasta and pastries, should be approached cautiously. They can be difficult to digest and may take up too much space in your stomach without offering much nutritional value. If you decide to try these foods, choose whole-grain options and introduce them in small amounts.

Hydration remains a key consideration during this phase, though the timing is just as crucial as the amount. Continue to separate drinking from eating, avoiding fluids during meals to prevent overfilling your stomach. Drinking too close to meal times can dilute digestive juices and lead to a feeling of bloating or discomfort. Instead, sip water or other sugar-free beverages throughout the day to maintain hydration without interfering with digestion.

The gradual reintroduction of solid foods is as much about listening to your body as it is about the food itself. Some days you might find that certain foods go down easily, while other days they don't sit quite right. That's part of the learning process. It's normal to have setbacks or to need to revisit softer foods if something doesn't agree with you. The goal is to build a varied diet that aligns with your nutritional needs and supports your long-term health. As you try different foods, take note of how they make you feel, adjusting your choices as necessary. The focus should always be on foods that provide the nourishment your body requires while being gentle enough for your new digestive system to handle comfortably.

This phase is about exploration and patience. You're learning to navigate a new way of eating, one that involves a careful balance of portions, textures and nutrients. With each meal, you're strengthening your relationship with food, transforming it into a source of enjoyment and nourishment rather than stress. By the end of this phase, you will have developed a deeper understanding of what your body needs and how to meet those needs in a way that supports your ongoing health and well-being.

Solid Recipes

❖

71. Soft Grilled Chicken Strips with Herbs

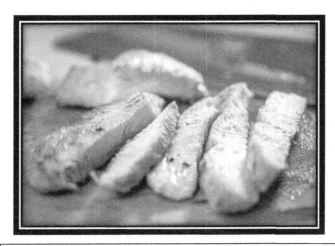

🔪 10 Min. 🕐 15 Min. 🍲 2 Serv. 👨‍🍳 Easy

Ingredients:
- 2 boneless, skinless chicken breasts
- 1 tbsp olive oil
- 1 tsp dried oregano
- 1 tsp garlic powder
- Salt and pepper to taste

Preparation:
1. Slice the chicken breasts into thin strips.
2. In a bowl, mix olive oil oregano, garlic powder, salt and pepper. Add the chicken strips and coat evenly.
3. Preheat a grill pan over medium heat. Grill the chicken strips for 3-4 minutes on each side until cooked through.
4. Serve warm with a side of soft vegetables if desired.

Comment: Tender and flavorful, these herb-seasoned chicken strips are a versatile option that pairs well with soft vegetables for a balanced and satisfying meal.

Nutritional info (per serving): Cal 180 | Carb 1g | Fat 8g | Prot 28g | Fib 0g.

72. Baked Salmon with Lemon and Dill

$\searchleftarrow$ 5 Min. $\quad \odot$ 15 Min. $\quad \lozenge$ 2 Serv. $\quad$ Easy

Ingredients:
- 2 salmon fillets (about 4 oz each)
- 1 tbsp lemon juice
- 1 tsp dried dill
- 1 tsp olive oil
- Salt and pepper to taste

Preparation:
1. Preheat the oven to 375°F (190°C).
2. Place the salmon fillets on a baking sheet lined with parchment paper. Drizzle with olive oil and lemon juice.
3. Sprinkle with dried dill, salt and pepper.
4. Bake for 12-15 minutes until the salmon is cooked through and flakes easily with a fork.

Comment: The delicate flavor of salmon is elevated by the freshness of dill and the brightness of lemon, creating a simple yet elegant dish packed with healthy fats.

Nutritional info (per serving): Cal 200 | Carb 1g | Fat 11g | Prot 24g | Fib 0g.

73. Tender Turkey Meatballs in Tomato Sauce

$\searchleftarrow$ 10 Min. $\quad \odot$ 20 Min. $\quad \lozenge$ 2 Serv. $\quad$ Medium

Ingredients:
- 1/2 lb ground turkey
- 1/4 cup breadcrumbs
- 1 egg
- 1 cup tomato sauce
- Salt and pepper to taste

Preparation:
1. In a bowl, mix the ground turkey, breadcrumbs, egg, salt and pepper. Form into small meatballs.
2. In a nonstick skillet, add the tomato sauce and bring to a simmer over medium heat.
3. Add the meatballs and cook for 15-20 minutes, turning occasionally, until the meatballs are cooked through.
4. Serve warm with a side of steamed vegetables.

Comment: These juicy turkey meatballs, simmered in a rich tomato sauce, offer a comforting and high-protein meal that's both flavorful and light.

Nutritional info (per serving): Cal 220 | Carb 10g | Fat 10g | Prot 24g | Fib 1g.

74. Soft Baked Cod with Garlic and Parsley

> 🔪 5 Min.   🕐 15 Min.   🍽 2 Serv.   👨‍🍳 Easy

Ingredients:
- 2 cod fillets (about 4 oz each)
- 1 tbsp olive oil
- 1 clove garlic, minced
- 1 tbsp fresh parsley, chopped
- Salt and pepper to taste

Preparation:
1. Preheat the oven to 375°F (190°C).
2. Place the cod fillets on a baking sheet lined with parchment paper. Drizzle with olive oil.
3. Sprinkle minced garlic, parsley, salt and pepper on top.
4. Bake for 12-15 minutes until the cod is cooked through and flakes easily with a fork.

Comment: Light and flaky cod fillets, enhanced with garlic and fresh parsley, deliver a dish that is both nourishing and subtly aromatic.

Nutritional info (per serving): Cal 150 | Carb 1g | Fat 7g | Prot 22g | Fib 0g.

75. Creamy Chicken Salad with Greek Yogurt

> 🔪 10 Min.   🕐 15 Min.   🍽 2 Serv.   👨‍🍳 Easy

Ingredients:
- 1 cup cooked chicken breast, shredded
- 1/4 cup plain Greek yogurt
- 1 tsp Dijon mustard
- 1/4 cup celery, finely chopped
- Salt and pepper to taste

Preparation:
1. In a bowl, combine the shredded chicken, Greek yogurt, Dijon mustard and celery.

2. Mix until the ingredients are well combined.
3. Season with salt and pepper to taste. Serve chilled.

Comment: This creamy chicken salad combines the tanginess of Greek yogurt with the crunch of celery, creating a light yet protein-packed dish that's perfect chilled.

Nutritional info (per serving): Cal 170 | Carb 3g | Fat 4g | Prot 28g | Fib 0g.

76. Stir-Fried Tofu with Soft Vegetables

🔪 10 Min. 🕐 10 Min. 🍲 2 Serv. 👨‍🍳 Easy

Ingredients:
- 1/2 block tofu, cubed
- 1 cup zucchini, sliced
- 1 tbsp soy sauce
- 1 tsp sesame oil
- 1 clove garlic, minced

Preparation:
1. In a nonstick skillet, heat the sesame oil over medium heat. Add the tofu cubes and stir-fry for 3-4 minutes until golden.
2. Add zucchini and minced garlic. Stir-fry for another 3-4 minutes until the vegetables are tender.
3. Drizzle with soy sauce and stir well before serving.

Comment: This vibrant stir-fry combines tender tofu with zucchini, soy sauce, and sesame oil, creating a dish that is as nutritious as it is flavorful.

Nutritional info (per serving): Cal 140 | Carb 7g | Fat 8g | Prot 10g | Fib 2g.

77. Avocado and Soft-Boiled Egg Salad

🔪 5 Min. 🕐 5 Min. 🍲 2 Serv. 👨‍🍳 Easy

Ingredients:
- 1 avocado, diced
- 2 large eggs
- 1 tbsp lemon juice
- Salt and pepper to taste
- 1 tbsp fresh chives, chopped

Preparation:

1. Bring a pot of water to a boil. Gently add eggs and cook for 4 minutes for a soft-boiled consistency.
2. Peel and chop the eggs. In a bowl, combine eggs with diced avocado.
3. Drizzle with lemon juice, salt and pepper. Garnish with fresh chives.

Comment: Creamy avocado and soft-boiled eggs come together in this refreshing salad, enhanced by a touch of lemon and a sprinkle of fresh chives for added zest.

Nutritional info (per serving): Cal 180 | Carb 6g | Fat 15g | Prot 7g | Fib 4g.

78. Zucchini Noodles with Marinara Sauce

> ✎ 10 Min. ⏱ 5 Min. 🍽 2 Serv. 👨‍🍳 Easy

Ingredients:

- 2 medium zucchinis, spiralized
- 1 cup marinara sauce
- 1 tbsp olive oil
- 1 clove garlic, minced
- Salt and pepper to taste

Preparation:

1. In a skillet, heat olive oil over medium heat. Add minced garlic and cook for 1 minute.
2. Add zucchini noodles and cook for 2-3 minutes until slightly softened.
3. Add marinara sauce, stir and cook for an additional 2 minutes. Season with salt and pepper before serving.

Comment: These light zucchini noodles, tossed with garlic and marinara sauce, are a flavorful and low-carb alternative to traditional pasta dishes.

Nutritional info (per serving): Cal 110 | Carb 10g | Fat 7g | Prot 3g | Fib 2g.

79. Soft Baked Eggplant with Tomato and Cheese

> ✎ 5 Min. ⏱ 15 Min. 🍽 2 Serv. 👨‍🍳 Easy

Ingredients:

- 1 medium eggplant, sliced
- 1/2 cup marinara sauce

- 1/4 cup shredded mozzarella cheese
- 1 tbsp olive oil
- Salt and pepper to taste

Preparation:

1. Preheat the oven to 375°F (190°C). Place eggplant slices on a baking sheet lined with parchment paper.
2. Drizzle with olive oil and season with salt and pepper. Bake for 10 minutes.
3. Remove from the oven, top with marinara sauce and mozzarella cheese. Return to the oven and bake for an additional 5 minutes until the cheese melts.

Comment: Baked eggplant slices topped with marinara sauce and melted mozzarella create a dish that is rich in flavor and ideal for a light yet satisfying meal.

Nutritional info (per serving): Cal 130 | Carb 10g | Fat 8g | Prot 5g | Fib 3g.

80. Chicken and Avocado Lettuce Wraps

✎ 10 Min. ⏱ 0 Min. 🍽 2 Serv. 👨‍🍳 Easy

Ingredients:

- 1 cup cooked chicken breast, shredded
- 1/2 avocado, diced
- 4 large lettuce leaves
- 1 tbsp lemon juice
- Salt and pepper to taste

Preparation:

1. In a bowl, combine the shredded chicken, diced avocado and lemon juice. Mix well.
2. Season with salt and pepper.
3. Spoon the mixture into lettuce leaves and serve as wraps.

Comment: These fresh and vibrant lettuce wraps, filled with shredded chicken and creamy avocado, offer a light and delicious meal with minimal preparation.

Nutritional info (per serving): Cal 180 | Carb 4g | Fat 10g | Prot 20g | Fib 2g.

81. Tender Turkey and Spinach Patties

🔪 10 Min.   ⏱ 10 Min.   🍽 2 Serv.   🍳 Medium

Ingredients:
- 1/2 lb ground turkey
- 1/2 cup fresh spinach, finely chopped
- 1 egg
- 1 clove garlic, minced
- Salt and pepper to taste

Preparation:
1. In a bowl, mix ground turkey, spinach, egg, garlic, salt and pepper. Form into small patties.
2. In a nonstick skillet, cook the patties over medium heat for 4-5 minutes on each side until cooked through.
3. Serve warm with a side of soft vegetables.

Comment: These turkey patties, enriched with fresh spinach, are juicy and high in protein, offering a flavorful yet light option for any meal.

Nutritional info (per serving): Cal 150 | Carb 2g | Fat 7g | Prot 20g | Fib 1g.

82. Soft Quinoa Salad with Avocado and Peas

🔪 10 Min.   ⏱ 15 Min.   🍽 2 Serv.   🍳 Medium

Ingredients:
- 1/2 cup quinoa
- 1 cup water
- 1/2 avocado, diced
- 1/4 cup peas
- 1 tbsp lemon juice

Preparation:
1. In a pot, bring water to a boil. Add quinoa, reduce heat and simmer for 10-12 minutes until tender.
2. Drain any excess water and let quinoa cool.
3. In a bowl, combine quinoa, avocado, peas and lemon juice. Mix well and serve.

Comment: The nutty quinoa, creamy avocado, and sweet peas combine in this refreshing salad, delivering a perfect balance of taste, texture, and nutrition.

Nutritional info (per serving): Cal 170 | Carb 22g | Fat 8g | Prot 5g | Fib 3g.

83. Mashed Chickpea and Veggie Bowl

> ✎ 10 Min. ⏱ 5 Min. 🍽 2 Serv. 👨‍🍳 Easy

Ingredients:
- 1/2 cup canned chickpeas, rinsed and drained
- 1/4 cup carrot, grated
- 1/4 cup cucumber, diced
- 1 tbsp olive oil
- Salt and pepper to taste

Preparation:
1. In a bowl, mash the chickpeas with a fork. Add grated carrot and diced cucumber.
2. Drizzle with olive oil and season with salt and pepper. Mix well.
3. Serve chilled or at room temperature.

Comment: This simple yet satisfying chickpea mash is elevated by fresh veggies and a drizzle of olive oil, creating a light and versatile dish.

Nutritional info (per serving): Cal 140 | Carb 16g | Fat 7g | Prot 5g | Fib 4g.

84. Oven-Baked Tilapia with Herbs

> ✎ 5 Min. ⏱ 15 Min. 🍽 2 Serv. 👨‍🍳 Easy

Ingredients:
- 2 tilapia fillets (about 4 oz each)
- 1 tbsp olive oil
- 1 tsp dried thyme
- 1 tsp garlic powder
- Salt and pepper to taste

Preparation:
1. Preheat the oven to 375°F (190°C). Place the tilapia fillets on a baking sheet lined with parchment paper.
2. Drizzle with olive oil and sprinkle with thyme, garlic powder, salt and pepper.
3. Bake for 12-15 minutes until the fish is cooked through and flakes easily.

Comment: Delicately seasoned with thyme and garlic, this oven-baked tilapia is a quick and healthy way to enjoy a protein-rich meal with minimal effort.

Nutritional info (per serving): Cal 160 | Carb 1g | Fat 8g | Prot 22g | Fib 0g.

85. Soft Cauliflower Rice Stir-Fry

🔪 10 Min.　🕐 10 Min.　🍳 2 Serv.　🗄 Easy

Ingredients:
- 2 cups cauliflower rice
- 1/2 cup peas
- 1 egg, beaten
- 1 tbsp soy sauce
- 1 tsp sesame oil

Preparation:
1. In a skillet, heat sesame oil over medium heat. Add the cauliflower rice and peas. Stir-fry for 5 minutes.
2. Push the mixture to the side of the pan and add the beaten egg. Scramble until cooked.
3. Mix everything together, add soy sauce and stir well before serving.

Comment: This light and flavorful stir-fry combines tender cauliflower rice and peas, enhanced with soy sauce and sesame oil for a quick, savory meal.

Nutritional info (per serving): Cal 110 | Carb 10g | Fat 5g | Prot 5g | Fib 3g.

86. Baked Sweet Potato with Cottage Cheese

🔪 5 Min.　🕐 30 Min.　🍳 2 Serv.　🗄 Easy

Ingredients:
- 1 medium sweet potato
- 1/2 cup cottage cheese
- 1/4 tsp cinnamon
- 1 tsp honey (optional)
- Salt to taste

Preparation:
1. Preheat the oven to 400°F (200°C). Wash the sweet potato and pierce it with a fork several times.

2. Place the sweet potato on a baking sheet and bake for 30 minutes or until tender.
3. Slice open the potato and top with cottage cheese, cinnamon and honey if desired. Sprinkle with salt before serving.

Comment: Sweet potato and creamy cottage cheese pair wonderfully in this dish, offering a perfect balance of natural sweetness and protein.

Nutritional info (per serving): Cal 150 | Carb 28g | Fat 2g | Prot 6g | Fib 4g.

87. Creamy Tuna Salad with Soft Veggies

✎ 10 Min. ⏲ 0 Min. ◍ 2 Serv. ⚙ Easy

Ingredients:
- 1 can tuna, drained
- 1/4 cup plain Greek yogurt
- 1/4 cup cucumber, finely diced
- 1 tbsp lemon juice
- Salt and pepper to taste

Preparation:
1. In a bowl, combine the drained tuna, Greek yogurt, cucumber and lemon juice.
2. Mix well until all ingredients are evenly coated.
3. Season with salt and pepper to taste. Serve chilled.

Comment: This creamy tuna salad is light yet packed with protein, complemented by the crisp freshness of finely diced cucumber.

Nutritional info (per serving): Cal 120 | Carb 3g | Fat 2g | Prot 23g | Fib 1g.

88. Soft Turkey and Vegetable Skillet

✎ 10 Min. ⏲ 15 Min. ◍ 2 Serv. ⚙ Medium

Ingredients:
- 1/2 lb ground turkey
- 1 cup zucchini, chopped
- 1/2 cup bell pepper, diced
- 1 tbsp olive oil
- Salt and pepper to taste

Preparation:

1. In a skillet, heat olive oil over medium heat. Add ground turkey and cook for 5 minutes until browned.
2. Add zucchini and bell pepper. Cook for an additional 7-8 minutes until vegetables are tender.
3. Season with salt and pepper to taste before serving.

Comment: Ground turkey and tender vegetables come together in this flavorful skillet dish, making it a wholesome and easy one-pan meal.

Nutritional info (per serving): Cal 200 | Carb 5g | Fat 10g | Prot 23g | Fib 2g.

89. Mashed Bean and Avocado Tacos

🔪 5 Min. ⏱ 5 Min. 🍽 2 Serv. 🪔 Easy

Ingredients:

- 1/2 cup canned black beans, rinsed and drained
- 1/2 avocado, mashed
- 2 small whole-grain tortillas
- 1 tsp lime juice
- Salt and pepper to taste

Preparation:

1. In a bowl, mash the black beans with the avocado and lime juice.
2. Season with salt and pepper to taste.
3. Spread the mixture onto the tortillas. Serve immediately.

Comment: These tacos combine creamy avocado and hearty black beans in whole-grain tortillas for a healthy and satisfying twist on a classic dish.

Nutritional info (per serving): Cal 180 | Carb 20g | Fat 9g | Prot 6g | Fib 5g.

90. Grilled Salmon with Mango Salsa

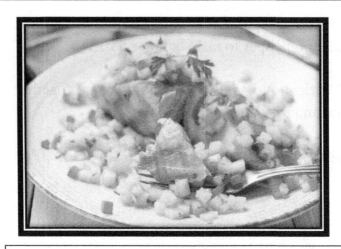

🔪 10 Min. 🕐 10 Min. 📷 2 Serv. 👨‍🍳 Medium

Ingredients:

- 2 salmon fillets (about 4 oz each)
- 1/2 cup mango, diced
- 1 tbsp lime juice
- 1 tbsp fresh cilantro, chopped
- Salt and pepper to taste

Preparation:

1. Preheat a grill or grill pan over medium heat.
2. Season the salmon fillets with salt and pepper. Grill for 4-5 minutes on each side until cooked through.
3. In a small bowl, mix diced mango, lime juice and cilantro.
4. Serve the grilled salmon topped with mango salsa.

Comment: The rich flavor of grilled salmon is perfectly balanced by the tropical sweetness of mango salsa, creating a vibrant and nutritious dish.

Nutritional info (per serving): Cal 220 | Carb 7g | Fat 12g | Prot 23g | Fib 1g.

91. Soft Baked Chicken and Zucchini Casserole

🔪 10 Min. 🕐 20 Min. 📷 2 Serv. 👨‍🍳 Medium

Ingredients:

- 1 cup cooked chicken breast, shredded
- 1 cup zucchini, grated

- 1/4 cup shredded mozzarella cheese
- 1 egg
- Salt and pepper to taste

Preparation:
1. Preheat the oven to 375°F (190°C).
2. In a bowl, combine shredded chicken, grated zucchini, mozzarella cheese and egg. Mix well.
3. Transfer the mixture to a greased baking dish. Bake for 20 minutes until the top is golden brown.
4. Season with salt and pepper to taste before serving.

Comment: This casserole combines tender chicken with the subtle freshness of zucchini and the creaminess of melted cheese, offering a balanced and satisfying meal that's easy to prepare.

Nutritional info (per serving): Cal 180 | Carb 3g | Fat 7g | Prot 24g | Fib 1g.

92. Quinoa and Soft Veggie Stuffed Peppers

🔪 10 Min. ⏱ 20 Min. 🍽 2 Serv. 🍳 Medium

Ingredients:
- 1/2 cup cooked quinoa
- 2 bell peppers, halved and seeded
- 1/4 cup zucchini, diced
- 1/4 cup tomato sauce
- Salt and pepper to taste

Preparation:
1. Preheat the oven to 375°F (190°C).
2. In a bowl, mix the cooked quinoa, diced zucchini and tomato sauce.
3. Stuff the bell pepper halves with the quinoa mixture.
4. Place the stuffed peppers on a baking sheet and bake for 20 minutes. Season with salt and pepper before serving.

Comment: Nutritious quinoa and tender zucchini come together inside sweet bell peppers, creating a visually appealing and wholesome dish rich in flavor and texture.

Nutritional info (per serving): Cal 140 | Carb 25g | Fat 2g | Prot 5g | Fib 4g.

93. Soft Spinach and Cheese Stuffed Chicken

✎ 10 Min. ⏱ 20 Min. 🍽 2 Serv. 👨‍🍳 Medium

Ingredients:
- 2 boneless chicken breasts
- 1/2 cup spinach, chopped
- 1/4 cup shredded mozzarella cheese
- 1 tbsp olive oil
- Salt and pepper to taste

Preparation:
1. Preheat the oven to 375°F (190°C).
2. Slice a pocket into each chicken breast. Stuff with spinach and mozzarella cheese.
3. In a skillet, heat olive oil over medium heat. Sear the chicken breasts for 3-4 minutes on each side.
4. Transfer the chicken to a baking dish and bake for 15 minutes until cooked through.

Comment: Juicy chicken breasts are filled with spinach and gooey mozzarella, creating a deliciously moist and protein-packed dish that's perfect for a special meal.

Nutritional info (per serving): Cal 220 | Carb 2g | Fat 10g | Prot 30g | Fib 1g.

94. Baked Cod with Spinach and Lemon

✎ 5 Min. ⏱ 15 Min. 🍽 2 Serv. 👨‍🍳 Easy

Ingredients:
- 2 cod fillets (about 4 oz each)
- 1 cup fresh spinach
- 1 tbsp lemon juice
- 1 tbsp olive oil
- Salt and pepper to taste

Preparation:
1. Preheat the oven to 375°F (190°C).
2. Place the cod fillets on a baking sheet lined with parchment paper. Arrange spinach leaves around the fillets.
3. Drizzle with lemon juice and olive oil. Season with salt and pepper.
4. Bake for 12-15 minutes until the cod is cooked through.

Comment: Flaky cod fillets are paired with fresh spinach and brightened by a drizzle of lemon, offering a light and flavorful entrée that's as healthy as it is easy to make.

Nutritional info (per serving): Cal 160 | Carb 2g | Fat 7g | Prot 23g | Fib 1g.

95. Tender Turkey Chili

✎ 10 Min. ⏱ 20 Min. 🍽 2 Serv. ⚗ Medium

Ingredients:
- 1/2 lb ground turkey
- 1 cup canned diced tomatoes
- 1/2 cup kidney beans, rinsed and drained
- 1 tbsp chili powder
- Salt to taste

Preparation:
1. In a pot, cook the ground turkey over medium heat until browned.
2. Add diced tomatoes, kidney beans and chili powder. Stir to combine.
3. Reduce heat and simmer for 15 minutes. Season with salt before serving.

Comment: This hearty turkey chili combines lean protein with beans and a touch of chili powder, creating a warm, comforting dish that's both nutritious and full of flavor.

Nutritional info (per serving): Cal 200 | Carb 18g | Fat 6g | Prot 22g | Fib 5g.

96. Soft Chicken and Cauliflower Bowl

✎ 10 Min. ⏱ 15 Min. 🍽 2 Serv. ⚗ Easy

Ingredients:
- 1 cup cooked chicken breast, diced
- 2 cups cauliflower florets
- 1 tbsp olive oil
- 1/2 tsp garlic powder
- Salt and pepper to taste

Preparation:
1. Steam cauliflower florets for about 10 minutes until tender.
2. In a skillet, heat olive oil over medium heat. Add cooked chicken and cauliflower.
3. Sprinkle with garlic powder, salt and pepper. Cook for 3-4 minutes until heated through.

Comment: Tender chicken and steamed cauliflower come together in this simple yet satisfying bowl, lightly seasoned with garlic for a flavorful and nutritious meal.

Nutritional info (per serving): Cal 180 | Carb 8g | Fat 7g | Prot 24g | Fib 3g.

97. Creamy Lentil and Spinach Salad

🔪 10 Min. ⏱ 15 Min. 🍽 2 Serv. 👨‍🍳 Easy

Ingredients:
- 1/2 cup cooked lentils
- 1 cup fresh spinach, chopped
- 1/4 cup plain Greek yogurt
- 1 tbsp lemon juice
- Salt and pepper to taste

Preparation:
1. In a bowl, combine the cooked lentils, chopped spinach, Greek yogurt and lemon juice.
2. Mix well until evenly coated.
3. Season with salt and pepper to taste. Serve immediately.

Comment: Protein-rich lentils and fresh spinach are combined with a creamy yogurt dressing, creating a vibrant and wholesome salad that's packed with nutrients and flavor.

Nutritional info (per serving): Cal 150 | Carb 25g | Fat 2g | Prot 10g | Fib 6g.

98. Avocado and Cucumber Sushi Rolls

🔪 10 Min. ⏱ 0 Min. 🍽 2 Serv. 👨‍🍳 Easy

Ingredients:
- 1/2 cup cooked sushi rice
- 1/2 avocado, sliced
- 1/4 cup cucumber, julienned
- 2 sheets nori
- 1 tbsp rice vinegar

Preparation:
1. Mix the cooked sushi rice with rice vinegar.
2. Place a sheet of nori on a flat surface. Spread half of the rice over the nori.

3. Arrange avocado slices and cucumber on top. Roll the nori tightly.
4. Slice into bite-sized pieces and serve.

Comment: These sushi rolls bring together creamy avocado and crisp cucumber for a refreshing and light dish, offering a perfect balance of textures and flavors.

Nutritional info (per serving): Cal 180 | Carb 28g | Fat 6g | Prot 3g | Fib 4g.

99. Soft Quinoa and Bean Stuffed Tomatoes

🔪 10 Min. ⏱ 15 Min. 🍽 2 Serv. 🍳 Medium

Ingredients:
- 2 medium tomatoes
- 1/2 cup cooked quinoa
- 1/4 cup canned black beans, rinsed and drained
- 1 tbsp olive oil
- Salt and pepper to taste

Preparation:
1. Preheat the oven to 375°F (190°C).
2. Slice the tops off the tomatoes and scoop out the seeds.
3. In a bowl, mix quinoa, black beans and olive oil. Season with salt and pepper.
4. Stuff the tomatoes with the quinoa mixture and bake for 15 minutes.

Comment: Juicy tomatoes are filled with a nutritious quinoa and bean mix, creating a delightful and colorful dish that's as visually appealing as it is wholesome.

Nutritional info (per serving): Cal 150 | Carb 20g | Fat 6g | Prot 4g | Fib 5g.

100. Grilled Shrimp with Avocado and Mango

🔪 10 Min. ⏱ 15 Min. 🍽 2 Serv. 🍳 Easy

Ingredients:
- 1/2 lb shrimp, peeled and deveined
- 1/2 avocado, diced
- 1/4 cup mango, diced
- 1 tbsp lime juice
- Salt and pepper to tast

Preparation:

1. Preheat a grill or grill pan over medium heat. Grill the shrimp for 2-3 minutes on each side until pink and cooked through.
2. In a bowl, mix diced avocado, mango and lime juice.
3. Serve the grilled shrimp topped with the avocado-mango mixture.

Comment: The sweetness of mango pairs beautifully with creamy avocado and tender grilled shrimp, making this dish a vibrant and nutrient-rich option for any meal.

Nutritional info (per serving): Cal 180 | Carb 10g | Fat 8g | Prot 20g | Fib 2g.

101. Soft Turkey Meatloaf with Carrots

✎ 10 Min. ⏱ 20 Min. 🍽 2 Serv. 🍴 Medium

Ingredients:

- 1/2 lb ground turkey
- 1/4 cup carrots, grated
- 1 egg
- 1 tbsp ketchup
- Salt and pepper to taste

Preparation:

1. Preheat the oven to 375°F (190°C).
2. In a bowl, mix the ground turkey, grated carrots, egg and ketchup.
3. Transfer the mixture to a small loaf pan and bake for 20 minutes until cooked through.

Comment: This tender turkey meatloaf, enriched with grated carrots for added moisture and sweetness, is a hearty and nutritious meal that's easy to prepare.

Nutritional info (per serving): Cal 170 | Carb 5g | Fat 6g | Prot 24g | Fib 1g.

102. Eggplant and Chicken Parmesan Bake

✎ 10 Min. ⏱ 20 Min. 🍽 2 Serv. 🍴 Medium

Ingredients:

- 1 cup cooked chicken breast, shredded
- 1 medium eggplant, sliced
- 1/2 cup marinara sauce
- 1/4 cup shredded mozzarella cheese

- Salt and pepper to taste

Preparation:
1. Preheat the oven to 375°F (190°C).
2. Layer eggplant slices, shredded chicken and marinara sauce in a baking dish.
3. Top with mozzarella cheese and bake for 20 minutes until the cheese is melted and bubbly.

Comment: Layers of eggplant, shredded chicken, and marinara sauce come together in this satisfying bake, topped with melted mozzarella for a comforting and protein-packed meal.

Nutritional info (per serving): Cal 180 | Carb 10g | Fat 8g | Prot 20g | Fib 3g.

103. Baked Chicken with Soft Asparagus

🔪 10 Min. 🕐 20 Min. 🍽 2 Serv. 👨‍🍳

Ingredients:
- 2 boneless chicken breasts
- 1 cup asparagus, trimmed
- 1 tbsp olive oil
- 1 clove garlic, minced
- Salt and pepper to taste

Preparation:
1. Preheat the oven to 375°F (190°C).
2. Place the chicken breasts and asparagus on a baking sheet. Drizzle with olive oil and sprinkle with minced garlic, salt and pepper.
3. Bake for 20 minutes until the chicken is cooked through.

Comment: Juicy chicken breasts are paired with tender asparagus and seasoned with garlic and olive oil, creating a simple, elegant, and nutritious dish.

Nutritional info (per serving): Cal 200 | Carb 4g | Fat 9g | Prot 28g | Fib 2g.

104. Soft Baked Tofu and Veggie Stir-Fry

🔪 10 Min. 🕐 10 Min. 🍽 2 Serv. 👨‍🍳 Easy

Ingredients:
- 1/2 block tofu, cubed
- 1/2 cup bell pepper, sliced

- 1/2 cup broccoli florets
- 1 tbsp soy sauce
- 1 tsp sesame oil

Preparation:
1. In a skillet, heat sesame oil over medium heat. Add the tofu and cook for 3-4 minutes until golden.
2. Add the bell pepper and broccoli. Stir-fry for another 5 minutes.
3. Drizzle with soy sauce and stir well before serving.

Comment: Golden tofu and fresh vegetables are stir-fried with sesame oil and soy sauce, delivering a dish that's light, flavorful, and packed with wholesome ingredients.

Nutritional info (per serving): Cal 140 | Carb 10g | Fat 7g | Prot 10g | Fib 3g.

105. Creamy Spinach and Mushroom Omelette

✎ 5 Min.   ⏱ 10 Min.   ◉ 2 Serv.   ⚖ Easy

Ingredients:
- 2 eggs
- 1/2 cup spinach, chopped
- 1/4 cup mushrooms, sliced
- 1 tbsp milk
- Salt and pepper to taste

Preparation:
1. In a bowl, beat the eggs with milk, salt and pepper.
2. In a nonstick skillet, cook the mushrooms over medium heat for 2 minutes until soft. Add spinach and cook for another 1 minute.
3. Pour the egg mixture over the vegetables. Cook for 3-4 minutes until the omelette is set. Fold in half and serve.

Comment: This fluffy omelette combines earthy mushrooms and fresh spinach for a balanced dish offering a creamy texture and a boost of protein to start your day.

Nutritional info (per serving): Cal 120 | Carb 3g | Fat 8g | Prot 10g | Fib 1g.

Chapter 5: Maintaining a Healthy Lifestyle

—————— ❖ ——————

Maintaining a healthy lifestyle after bariatric surgery is about creating a balanced approach to daily habits that support your physical and mental well-being. It's not just about following a strict diet or exercise routine but finding a rhythm that fits seamlessly into your life. By embracing meal planning, learning to manage cravings and incorporating physical activity, you build a foundation for long-term success. This phase is where the work you've put into adapting your diet and mindset comes together, empowering you to live fully and enjoy the benefits of your journey.

Meal Planning and Managing Cravings

Maintaining a healthy lifestyle post-surgery revolves around thoughtful meal planning and understanding how to manage cravings. After all the work you've put into adapting to your new way of eating, meal planning becomes the backbone of staying on track. It's about finding a rhythm that suits your life and ensures that each meal meets your body's needs. Planning meals ahead of time helps you avoid the pitfalls of impulsive choices and keeps you focused on nourishing yourself in a balanced, intentional way.

A good starting point is to carve out some time each week to plan your meals. Think about what you'll need for breakfast, lunch, dinner and snacks, making sure to include a variety of foods that provide protein, fiber and essential nutrients. Having a game plan reduces the stress of last-minute decisions, making it easier to stick to your dietary goals. A well-stocked kitchen with the right ingredients is your ally, so make a habit of creating a grocery list that aligns with your planned meals. This doesn't mean your meals need to be complex or time-consuming. Simplicity often works best. Preparing easy-to-digest, nutritious options like a batch of quinoa salad, grilled chicken or roasted vegetables ensures you have go-to meals ready when hunger strikes.

Portion control is equally important. Use measuring cups or a food scale when preparing your meals to keep portions in check. Your stomach's capacity remains smaller, so focusing on smaller, frequent meals is key to avoiding discomfort and ensuring you get the right amount of nutrients throughout the day. It's helpful to pack meals in small containers, especially if you're on the go, so you're not tempted to overeat. Taking the time to portion meals in advance makes it easier to maintain your balance and prevents the impulse to grab whatever is available when hunger hits.

Managing cravings is another essential part of maintaining your lifestyle. Cravings are natural and can be triggered by stress, boredom or even habit. The goal isn't to eliminate cravings altogether but to understand them and respond in a way that aligns with your health goals. When a craving strikes, take a moment to ask yourself if you're truly hungry or if something else might be driving that urge.

Sometimes, sipping water or engaging in a different activity can help shift the focus away from food. If it's genuine hunger, aim for a satisfying snack that combines protein and fiber, like a small portion of Greek yogurt with berries or a handful of nuts. These choices help curb hunger without derailing your progress.

Having healthy alternatives readily available is crucial for managing cravings effectively. Stock your pantry and fridge with options that satisfy your taste buds without compromising your nutrition. If you have a sweet tooth, keeping fruit or sugar-free gelatin on hand can offer a naturally sweet treat. For savory cravings, try things like hummus with sliced veggies or a small serving of low-fat cheese. These choices are satisfying, yet still align with your dietary needs, making it easier to resist reaching for high-calorie, low-nutrient snacks.

Preparation is your secret weapon against cravings. Cooking meals ahead of time and having them readily available reduces the likelihood of impulsive eating. When you have a craving, knowing that you have a prepped, nutritious option can make all the difference. Consider batch-cooking soups, stews or grilled proteins at the start of the week. Then, portion them into containers that are easy to grab when you need a meal or snack. This kind of foresight gives you control and empowers you to make choices that support your goals.

Mindful eating also plays a key role in managing cravings. Take the time to enjoy each meal, savoring the flavors and textures. Eating slowly allows you to tune into your body's signals of fullness and satisfaction, helping you recognize when you've had enough. This practice not only aids in digestion but also enhances your awareness of what truly satisfies your hunger. It's easy to mistake a craving for hunger when you eat quickly or while distracted. By making mealtime an intentional and enjoyable experience, you strengthen your ability to distinguish between a physical need for food and a fleeting desire for something specific.

Cravings can also be reduced by adding variety to your meals. Eating the same foods repeatedly can lead to boredom, which often triggers the desire for something new or different. Experiment with spices, herbs and new recipes to keep your meals interesting and flavorful. Trying different proteins, vegetables and whole grains not only makes eating more enjoyable but also ensures that you're getting a range of nutrients that keep your body satisfied.

Maintaining a healthy lifestyle isn't about perfection; it's about consistency and balance. Meal planning and managing cravings are part of the long-term strategy to support your success. They help you stay mindful of your choices and create a positive relationship with food that goes beyond simply fueling your body. By taking the time to plan and prepare, you're setting yourself up for a lifestyle that is not only healthy but also sustainable and satisfying.

Physical Activity and Long-Term Weight Management

Incorporating physical activity into your daily routine is essential for maintaining a healthy lifestyle after bariatric surgery. It's not just about burning calories; it's about building strength, boosting energy and enhancing your overall sense of well-being. The way your body processes food and stores energy has changed and exercise is a powerful tool to support these new dynamics. Movement helps you preserve muscle mass, improve metabolism and keep the weight off in the long run.

Getting started with physical activity may feel daunting, especially if exercise wasn't a regular part of your life before surgery. The key is to approach it gradually and with compassion for where you are in your journey. Right now, your goal is to find movement that feels good and is sustainable. It's not about pushing your limits immediately but rather about integrating activity into your routine in a way that becomes a natural and enjoyable part of your lifestyle.

Begin with low-impact exercises, particularly if you're still in the early stages of recovery. Walking is an excellent place to start. It's gentle on the joints, requires no special equipment and can be done almost anywhere. Start with short, manageable walks, maybe just around your neighborhood or even indoors if the weather isn't cooperating. The important part is to get moving, allowing your body to adjust and gradually increase stamina. As you build up strength and confidence, extend your walking time or add light inclines to challenge yourself a bit more. Even small steps like parking farther from the store or taking the stairs can make a significant difference over time.

Once you feel more comfortable, consider incorporating a variety of exercises to keep things interesting. Activities like swimming, cycling, yoga or light strength training offer diverse ways to engage different muscle groups and enhance flexibility. Swimming, in particular, is fantastic for those looking for a low-impact, full-body workout that doesn't put pressure on the joints. Yoga can help improve balance, increase flexibility and reduce stress, adding a mindful component to your physical activity routine. Strength training, using light weights or resistance bands, is crucial for maintaining and building muscle mass. After bariatric surgery, muscle mass can decrease due to rapid weight loss, so incorporating some form of resistance training helps to counteract that loss and boosts your metabolism.

Staying active doesn't mean spending hours at the gym. Consistency matters more than intensity, especially at the beginning. Aim to integrate movement into your daily life in ways that feel enjoyable and manageable. Maybe it's a dance class, gardening or playing a sport you love. The best kind of exercise is the one you enjoy enough to stick with, so experiment until you find activities that make you feel energized and uplifted. Engaging in something you genuinely like will make it easier to commit to regular exercise, turning it into a habit rather than a chore.

Long-term weight management is not just about the physical effort but also about finding balance and joy in movement. Set small, achievable goals and celebrate each milestone you reach. As you gain strength and stamina, you'll notice how physical activity positively affects your mood, energy levels and sleep quality. This holistic improvement reinforces the benefits of staying active, motivating you to continue as part of your healthy lifestyle.

Accountability can be a powerful motivator. Finding a workout buddy, joining a fitness class or participating in an online community can provide encouragement and support. When you connect with others who are on a similar path, it creates a sense of camaraderie and can make exercising more fun. Whether it's a weekly yoga class with a friend or a walking group in your neighborhood, having a support system makes it easier to stay committed to your activity goals.

Listening to your body is crucial throughout this process. Some days will feel easier than others and it's important to honor your body's signals. Rest and recovery are just as important as the activity itself. Overexertion can lead to injury or burnout, so pay attention to how your body responds to different forms of exercise. Incorporate rest days and gentle activities like stretching or meditation to give your body the recovery time it needs to stay healthy and strong.

Living a healthy lifestyle post-surgery is an ongoing process that involves commitment, mindfulness and flexibility. Through consistent meal planning, managing cravings thoughtfully and making physical activity a regular part of your life, you equip yourself to meet your long-term health goals. Every small step you take toward nourishing your body and staying active strengthens the foundation for a sustainable, fulfilling lifestyle. Embrace this path, knowing that it's about more than just weight management, it's about enhancing your quality of life and enjoying each moment with renewed energy and confidence.

The Role of Sleep and Stress Management

Achieving a balanced lifestyle after bariatric surgery goes beyond diet and exercise; restful sleep and effective stress management are equally crucial for sustaining your health and overall well-being. Sleep affects almost every aspect of health, from metabolism and immune function to mental clarity and emotional resilience. After surgery, getting sufficient rest becomes even more essential as your body undergoes a period of intense healing and adjustment. In parallel, managing stress is vital, as stress can undermine efforts to maintain a balanced lifestyle and lead to cravings, overeating or other behaviors that might derail your progress. Together, sleep and stress management serve as pillars for long-term health, helping you feel energized, focused and more in control of your journey.

Quality sleep supports the body's healing process, regulates hunger cues and maintains steady energy levels throughout the day. When you don't get enough rest, your body produces more hunger hormones, like ghrelin, which can intensify hunger even when your body has sufficient nourishment. Lack of sleep can lead to fatigue, making it harder to stay committed to healthy eating habits, resist cravings and feel motivated to engage in physical activity. Additionally, poor sleep can affect concentration, mood and overall quality of life, leading to irritability, low energy and difficulty focusing on personal goals.

For most people, the ideal sleep range is between seven and nine hours per night, which generally promotes the best health outcomes. Developing a calming bedtime routine – such as reading, meditating or doing gentle stretches – can help prepare your body for rest, improving both the quality and consistency of your sleep. Creating a sleep-friendly environment by keeping the bedroom cool, dark and quiet also supports better rest. Avoiding screens and large meals before bed helps reduce mental and digestive stimulation, making it easier to fall asleep and stay asleep.

Stress management is equally important in your post-surgery lifestyle. Stress is a natural part of life, but chronic stress can lead to spikes in cortisol, a hormone that, when elevated for extended periods, can disrupt metabolism and increase cravings for high-sugar or high-fat foods. Learning to recognize the signs of stress and developing healthy ways to cope can significantly impact your long-term success. Identifying stressors in your daily life is a valuable first step; once you understand what causes stress, you can start creating strategies to address or minimize it.

Practicing mindfulness or deep breathing techniques can be an effective way to relieve stress in the moment. Taking a few minutes each day to focus on slow, controlled breathing or a guided meditation helps lower cortisol levels, creating a sense of calm and focus. Even small changes, like taking regular breaks during the day or spending a few minutes outdoors, can have a positive effect on your overall stress levels.

Physical activity also plays a role in stress management. Exercise releases endorphins, natural mood boosters that help reduce stress and improve mood. Engaging in activities you enjoy, whether it's walking, yoga or dancing, can be an excellent way to let go of tension. Movement not only benefits your physical health but also provides an emotional release, offering a constructive outlet for stress and helping you feel more balanced. Additionally, engaging in activities that bring you joy and fulfillment, such as hobbies, spending time with loved ones or practicing relaxation techniques, can create a sense of calm and satisfaction that offsets daily stressors.

Support systems can also be invaluable for managing stress. Connecting with others who understand your journey – whether friends, family or members of a support group – can provide encouragement, perspective and a listening ear when you need it most. Sometimes, simply talking through challenges can make them feel more manageable. Consider reaching out to a therapist or counselor if stress feels overwhelming, as they can offer tools to help you navigate difficult emotions and create coping strategies tailored to your situation.

Finding balance between sleep, stress management and other healthy lifestyle habits creates a positive feedback loop, where each element reinforces the other. Good sleep enhances your ability to cope with stress, while effective stress management improves sleep quality. Together, they strengthen your body's resilience, making it easier to maintain your dietary goals, stay active and fully enjoy the benefits of your post-surgery lifestyle.

Remember that sleep and stress management are not just supplementary but foundational to your well-being. By prioritizing these elements, you're building a strong base for sustained health, empowering yourself to face challenges with resilience and pursue each day with renewed energy and confidence.

Chapter 6: Additional Resources

---　❖　---

Shopping Lists

Fresh and Nourishing Vegetables

Fill your cart with vegetables that blend easily, can be cooked to a soft consistency and are packed with nutrients. Choose:

- Spinach, kale and Swiss chard for smoothies, soups and purees.
- Broccoli, cauliflower, zucchini and carrots for mashing, blending or roasting.
- Butternut squash, sweet potatoes and pumpkin for creamy soups and purees.
- Leeks, tomatoes and beets for light broths and blended soups.

These vegetables provide essential vitamins, minerals and fiber, promoting digestion and aiding in the body's recovery process.

Lean Protein Sources

Select proteins that are easily digestible and can be prepared in soft or blended forms:

- Skinless poultry (chicken or turkey breast) for soft casseroles, broths and purees.
- Fresh fish (salmon, tilapia, cod) to flake into soft dishes or soups.
- Tofu and silken tofu for smoothies, mashes and stir-fries.
- Eggs for soft scrambles, purees and high-protein meals.
- Lentils, chickpeas and beans for creamy soups, mashes and nutritious purees.
- Greek yogurt and low-fat cottage cheese for parfaits, smoothies and creamy blends.

Grains and Fiber-Rich Options

Whole grains provide energy and aid in digestion. Stock up on:

- Quinoa and couscous for light mashes and salads.
- Rolled oats for smoothies and pureed breakfast options.
- Cream of rice or wheat cereals for easy-to-digest breakfast choices.
- Brown rice for soft stir-fries and gentle grain salads.

Healthy Fats and Oils

Incorporate fats that are essential for healing and nutrient absorption:

- Avocados for mashing, blending with cottage cheese or adding to smoothies.
- Extra virgin olive oil for cooking and drizzling over pureed soups or salads.
- Nuts (such as almonds, walnuts) and seeds (chia, flaxseeds) to add to smoothies, chia puddings or yogurt blends.
- Nut butters (like peanut or almond butter) for smoothies and protein-rich snacks.

Fruit for Flavor and Nutrients:ì
Choose fruits that can be blended or mashed for a variety of dishes:
- Bananas, apples, pears and peaches for smoothies, purees and soft desserts.
- Berries (strawberries, blueberries, raspberries) for smoothies, chia puddings and yogurt parfaits.
- Citrus fruits (oranges, lemons) for adding zest and flavor to broths, soups and smoothies.
- Soft, ripe mangoes for tropical smoothies and purees.

Dairy and Alternatives
Opt for low-fat, easy-to-digest options that provide protein and calcium:
- Greek yogurt (plain, low-fat) for smoothies, parfaits and creamy purees.
- Low-fat milk or plant-based milk alternatives (almond, soy, coconut) for blending with soups, smoothies and puddings.
- Low-fat cottage cheese for mashing with avocado or incorporating into soft salads.

Herbs, Spices and Flavor Enhancers
Enhance the taste of your meals without relying on salt or sugar:
- Fresh herbs like parsley, cilantro, rosemary and thyme for garnishing soups and soft dishes.
- Spices such as cinnamon, turmeric, ginger and nutmeg for adding warmth and flavor to soups, smoothies and purees.
- Garlic and onion for soups, broths and mashes to boost flavor naturally.

Hydration and Beverages
Staying hydrated is crucial:
- Herbal teas (chamomile, peppermint) for soothing beverages.
- Coconut water and electrolyte-infused drinks for hydration during the early phases.
- Unsweetened almond milk, soy milk or oat milk for smoothies and light soups.

Omega-3-Rich Foods
Prioritize these for their healing benefits:
- Fresh fish like salmon, mackerel or trout for baking, steaming or blending into soft dishes.
- Chia seeds and flaxseeds to mix into smoothies, puddings or yogurt.

Snack Options
Prepare for those in-between meal moments with snacks that align with your diet:
- Greek yogurt with honey or fruit for a satisfying, protein-rich snack.
- Soft boiled eggs or egg-based dishes for a quick, nutritious bite.
- Small portions of avocado mash or cottage cheese with fruit for a balanced snack.

28-Day Meal Plan

Day	Breakfast	Lunch	Dinner	Snack	Dessert
1	Blended Oatmeal Smoothie	Creamy Pumpkin Soup	Creamy Chicken Broth	Cucumber Mint Cooler	Classic Gazpacho (Blended)
2	Berry Protein Shake	Carrot-Ginger Soup	Savory Bone Broth Elixir	Watermelon Coconut Drink	Silky Zucchini Soup
3	Green Detox Shake	Smooth Cauliflower Soup	Protein-Packed Vegetable Broth	Golden Turmeric Milk	Broccoli and Cheese Soup
4	Peanut Butter Banana Smoothie	Butternut Squash Soup	Classic Miso Soup	Coconut Curry Broth	Smooth Beet Soup
5	Creamy Chia Seed Shake	Tomato Basil Soup	Zesty Lemon Chicken Soup	Savory Egg Drop Soup	Sweet Potato Coconut Soup
6	Strawberry Kefir Smoothie	Light Spinach and Leek Soup	Silky Mushroom Soup	Creamy Celery Soup	Silken Tofu and Spinach Soup
7	Tropical Mango Smoothie	Creamy Pea Soup	Smooth Potato and Chive Soup	Green Pea and Mint Soup	Apple Cinnamon Protein Shake
8	Soft Scrambled Eggs with Cheese	Savory Ricotta and Herb Mash	Creamy Mashed Cauliflower	Soft Tofu and Berry Parfait	Soft Banana and Greek Yogurt Blend
9	Smooth Cottage Cheese and Avocado Mix	Mashed Sweet Potato Delight	Silky Pumpkin Puree	Smooth Apple-Cinnamon Oatmeal	Silky Carrot and Ginger Mash
10	Smooth Apple-Cinnamon Oatmeal	Blended Chickpea and Tahini Puree	Soft Baked Apple and Cinnamon Mix	Ricotta and Spinach Puree	Creamy Rice Pudding with Nutmeg
11	Greek Yogurt and Honey Swirl	Creamy Butternut Squash and Carrot Blend	Creamy Spinach and Ricotta Blend	Smooth Zucchini and Potato Blend	Silken Tofu with Honey and Vanilla
12	Mango Chia Seed Pudding	Soft Pea and Mint Mash	Mashed Cauliflower and Cheddar Blend	Smooth Sweet Potato and Cinnamon Mix	Soft Baked Apple and Cinnamon Mix

13	Soft Banana and Greek Yogurt Blend	Mashed Black Beans and Avocado	Blended Chicken and Broccoli Mash	Mashed Avocado with Soft-Boiled Egg	Smooth Sweet Potato and Cinnamon Mix
14	Silken Tofu with Honey and Vanilla	Creamy Pumpkin and Quinoa Mash	Soft Cottage Cheese with Peaches	Creamy Polenta with Parmesan	Mango Chia Seed Pudding
15	Creamy Spinach and Mushroom Omelette	Tender Turkey Meatballs in Tomato Sauce	Soft Grilled Chicken Strips with Herbs	Mashed Chickpea and Veggie Bowl	Creamy Mashed Cauliflower
16	Soft Quinoa Salad with Avocado and Peas	Soft Baked Eggplant with Tomato and Cheese	Soft Turkey and Vegetable Skillet	Soft Cottage Cheese with Peaches	Soft Cottage Cheese with Peaches
17	Avocado and Soft-Boiled Egg Salad	Chicken and Avocado Lettuce Wraps	Soft Baked Chicken and Zucchini Casserole	Soft Baked Chicken and Zucchini Casserole	Soft Banana and Greek Yogurt Blend
18	Baked Salmon with Lemon and Dill	Soft Quinoa Salad with Avocado and Peas	Soft Quinoa and Bean Stuffed Tomatoes	Creamy Tuna Salad with Soft Veggies	Blended Oatmeal Smoothie
19	Creamy Chicken Salad with Greek Yogurt	Mashed Chickpea and Veggie Bowl	Soft Turkey Meatloaf with Carrots	Soft Grilled Chicken Strips with Herbs	Soft Pea and Mint Mash
20	Soft Grilled Chicken Strips with Herbs	Oven-Baked Tilapia with Herbs	Soft Baked Tofu and Veggie Stir-Fry	Tender Turkey Chili	Creamy Pumpkin and Quinoa Mash
21	Stir-Fried Tofu with Soft Vegetables	Soft Cauliflower Rice Stir-Fry	Baked Cod with Spinach and Lemon	Baked Salmon with Lemon and Dill	Smooth Apple-Cinnamon Oatmeal
22	Zucchini Noodles with Marinara Sauce	Baked Sweet Potato with Cottage Cheese	Eggplant and Chicken Parmesan Bake	Soft Grilled Chicken Strips with Herbs	Creamy Chicken Salad with Greek Yogurt
23	Soft Turkey and Spinach Patties	Grilled Salmon with Mango Salsa	Soft Grilled Chicken Strips with Herbs	Creamy Spinach and Mushroom Omelette	Soft Cottage Cheese with Peaches

24	Soft Quinoa and Bean Stuffed Tomatoes	Soft Spinach and Cheese Stuffed Chicken	Soft Turkey and Vegetable Skillet	Soft Turkey Meatloaf with Carrots	Soft Banana and Greek Yogurt Blend
25	Creamy Tuna Salad with Soft Veggies	Tender Turkey Chili	Creamy Lentil and Spinach Salad	Soft Baked Tofu and Veggie Stir-Fry	Silken Tofu with Honey and Vanilla
26	Eggplant and Chicken Parmesan Bake	Soft Chicken and Cauliflower Bowl	Avocado and Cucumber Sushi Rolls	Avocado and Cucumber Sushi Rolls	Smooth Sweet Potato and Cinnamon Mix
27	Baked Chicken with Soft Asparagus	Grilled Shrimp with Avocado and Mango	Soft Quinoa Salad with Avocado and Peas	Soft Quinoa Salad with Avocado and Peas	Mango Chia Seed Pudding
28	Soft Cottage Cheese with Peaches	Soft Grilled Chicken Strips with Herbs	Soft Cottage Cheese with Peaches	Creamy Rice Pudding with Nutmeg	Soft Baked Apple and Cinnamon Mix

Conclusion

—— ❖ ——

Reaching this point is a testament to your journey of transformation and commitment to a healthier lifestyle. Bariatric surgery was the starting line, but the changes you've embraced since then have laid the foundation for a new way of living. From redefining your relationship with food to incorporating mindful eating and physical activity, every step has contributed to your progress. This journey is not about reaching a finish line but about continuously nurturing your well-being and adapting to your body's evolving needs. It's a path of empowerment, learning and self-care that shapes your future.

Final Reflections and Supporting Resources

Reflecting on the journey you've embarked on, it's clear that life after bariatric surgery is more than just a change in eating habits; it's a holistic transformation. This path is about nurturing your body and mind, learning new ways to relate to food and embracing habits that promote long-term health. It's not a quick fix, but rather an ongoing process of self-discovery and adaptation. By now, you've navigated through various phases of eating, listened to your body's cues and developed strategies to support your well-being. This growth represents a profound commitment to taking control of your health and living life more fully.

Surgery may have been the catalyst for this change, but it's the daily choices you make that shape the lasting impact on your health. Each phase, each meal, each moment of mindful eating has been a building block in creating a lifestyle that suits your new reality. What you've done is lay the groundwork for a future where food is not a source of stress but a means to nourish and energize. It's important to acknowledge this progress and to be kind to yourself during this ongoing journey. There will be ups and downs, successes and setbacks, but each experience is an opportunity to learn and adjust.

One of the most significant reflections to take away from this experience is the value of mindfulness. Whether it's planning meals, managing cravings or engaging in physical activity, being present in these moments helps you connect with your body's needs. This awareness allows you to make choices that align with your health goals, bringing a sense of intention and balance into your daily routine. Mindfulness isn't about perfection; it's about paying attention to what your body is telling you and responding in a way that supports your overall well-being.

It's also worth noting that this journey is deeply personal. No two paths are the same and comparing your progress to others can be both misleading and disheartening. Your body has unique needs and preferences and learning what works best for you is key. What matters most is that you've committed to this path and continue to make choices that prioritize your health. As time goes on, you'll likely continue to fine-tune your diet and exercise habits, finding what brings you both physical comfort and joy. Embrace this individuality and give yourself the freedom to explore new foods, activities and routines that fit into your evolving lifestyle.

Supporting resources play a crucial role in helping you maintain this lifestyle. While you've gained a wealth of knowledge about nutrition, meal planning and physical activity, it's natural to seek additional guidance along the way. Staying connected with your healthcare team is invaluable; they provide professional advice tailored to your progress and can help you navigate any challenges that arise. Regular check-ups offer an opportunity to monitor your health, adjust your dietary needs and discuss any concerns you may have.

In addition to medical support, seeking out community resources can provide a sense of connection and motivation. Local support groups or online forums dedicated to bariatric patients offer a space to share experiences, exchange tips and find encouragement. Knowing that others are walking a similar path can be comforting and empowering, reminding you that you're not alone in this process. These communities can provide fresh perspectives, introduce new recipes or even recommend products that align with your dietary needs. Being part of such a network enriches your journey and reinforces your commitment to a healthier lifestyle.

Educational resources are equally important. Continuing to learn about nutrition, cooking techniques and mindful eating practices keeps you informed and inspired. Cookbooks, reputable websites and even cooking classes can expand your repertoire and keep meals exciting. Variety is key to maintaining a balanced diet, so exploring new foods and preparation methods helps prevent boredom and keeps you engaged in your healthy routine.

Lastly, never underestimate the power of self-care as a supporting resource. Taking time to nurture your mental and emotional health is just as vital as caring for your physical body. Whether it's through meditation, journaling or simply taking a walk in nature, self-care practices help you reconnect with your goals and recharge your motivation. Remember, this journey is not just about what you eat but about fostering a lifestyle that supports every aspect of your well-being.

Moving forward, the most important thing is to stay adaptable. Your body will continue to change and your lifestyle may evolve with new routines, tastes and needs. This flexibility is a strength, allowing you to adjust as you learn more about what makes you feel your best. Use the tools, strategies and knowledge you've gained to keep steering yourself toward a balanced, nourishing way of living. Every day is an opportunity to take another step on this path, reinforcing your commitment to a healthier, more fulfilling life.

Celebrating Milestones and Progress

Reflecting on how far you've come is an essential part of maintaining motivation and appreciating the progress you've made. Bariatric surgery was just the beginning, but the real achievements lie in each small victory you've accumulated along the way. Every milestone, whether it's adjusting to new eating habits, successfully navigating social situations or discovering physical activities that bring you joy, represents a significant step toward a healthier lifestyle. Recognizing and celebrating these moments reinforces your commitment to change, giving you the confidence to keep moving forward.

Celebrations don't need to be grand gestures; sometimes, the most meaningful milestones are the personal ones that may go unnoticed by others. Perhaps you've mastered meal planning or you've reached a fitness goal that once seemed out of reach. Taking a moment to acknowledge these achievements can create a positive feedback loop, where each accomplishment strengthens your desire to maintain a balanced lifestyle. Setting personal goals and noting your progress can help make these accomplishments more tangible, serving as reminders of your resilience and dedication. Tracking your progress is one way to celebrate your journey. Consider keeping a journal where you document your experiences, note changes in your energy levels or reflect on how your mindset has shifted since the beginning. Reading over these entries can be a powerful way to see just how much you've accomplished and to remind yourself of the hard work and patience that have brought you here. If you're inclined, taking photos or recording measurements at different points in your journey can also provide visual evidence of your progress, reinforcing the positive impact of your lifestyle changes.

Milestones aren't only about physical changes; they encompass mental and emotional growth as well. Each time you resist an old habit, manage a craving with mindfulness or approach a meal with gratitude rather than stress, you're strengthening your mental resilience. These are major victories that deserve recognition. Celebrate these moments by doing something that brings you joy, whether it's a small reward like treating yourself to a new book or taking a day to enjoy your favorite hobby. Recognizing these changes reinforces your dedication to a healthier mindset, encouraging you to stay committed.

Involving loved ones in your milestones can make celebrations even more meaningful. Sharing your progress with friends, family or members of a support group allows others to see your hard work and provides an additional layer of encouragement. Whether it's a conversation over coffee, a walk with a friend or sharing a meal you've prepared, these shared moments offer a sense of connection and recognition from those who care about your journey. Celebrating with others reminds you that you're not alone and that your progress is something worth honoring.

As you continue along this path, remember that every milestone, no matter how small, is a testament to your strength, perseverance and commitment. Celebrating these achievements isn't just a reward it's an affirmation of the lifestyle you're building. By acknowledging the steps you've taken, you're cultivating a sense of pride and gratitude that reinforces your motivation. These celebrations are not the end of your journey but joyful pauses that highlight just how much you've grown, encouraging you to keep moving forward with confidence and purpose.

STAYING MOTIVATED FOR LIFELONG SUCCESS

Maintaining motivation over the long term is essential for sustaining the healthy lifestyle you've worked so hard to establish. Motivation can ebb and flow, especially as the initial excitement of change evolves into the everyday commitment required for lasting success. Staying motivated means continuously reconnecting with your "why" – the reasons you embarked on this journey in the first place. This clarity provides the foundation for your progress, reminding you of the value these changes bring to your life and helping you stay focused even on challenging days.

One of the most powerful ways to maintain motivation is to set new, evolving goals that align with where you are in your journey. After bariatric surgery, your initial goals may have focused on immediate recovery and adjusting to a new eating routine. As you progress, creating fresh goals keeps you engaged and prevents stagnation. Perhaps you'll aim to expand your physical activities, experiment with new recipes or deepen your practice of mindful eating. These evolving targets give you something tangible to work toward, helping you stay connected to your journey's purpose.

Variety is another key to sustaining motivation. Trying new activities, exploring different foods and finding fresh ways to enjoy your routine can keep things interesting and prevent feelings of monotony. Explore new types of movement that feel enjoyable, like dancing, hiking or trying a fitness class. In the kitchen, experiment with seasonal produce, explore different cuisines or try cooking techniques that keep meals exciting. Maintaining flexibility in your approach allows you to adapt to your changing tastes and interests, which makes sticking to your routine more enjoyable and sustainable.

Building a support system also plays an essential role in staying motivated. Connecting with others who are on a similar path – whether through support groups, social media communities or simply friends and family who encourage your lifestyle – can provide a sense of camaraderie and accountability. Sharing both achievements and challenges with a supportive network helps you feel understood and less isolated. Being part of a community reinforces your commitment and seeing others' progress can be inspiring, reminding you of your own potential for growth.

Maintaining a positive mindset is equally vital. The road to lasting success isn't always straightforward; there will be highs and lows and moments when motivation wanes. In these instances, practicing self-compassion can help you move forward without getting discouraged. Accept that setbacks are a natural part of any journey and rather than seeing them as failures, view them as opportunities to learn and adjust. Being kind to yourself during these moments fosters resilience, helping you stay focused on the big picture rather than getting bogged down by temporary obstacles.

A simple but effective strategy to reignite motivation is to regularly revisit the progress you've made. Reflecting on how much your health, energy and mindset have changed can be an empowering reminder of why you began this journey. Celebrate small victories and acknowledge the hard work you've put in to reach each new stage. These reflections not only reinforce your dedication but also give you a sense of pride in what you've achieved, making it easier to stay committed to your goals. Finally, keep in mind that motivation doesn't always have to be at its peak for you to stay on track.

Building consistent habits that support your health can help carry you through days when motivation may be lower. Establishing a routine with regular meal planning, setting aside time for movement and practicing mindfulness ensures that these habits become second nature, reducing the reliance on willpower alone. In this way, motivation becomes a supportive force rather than a constant requirement, allowing you to navigate your journey with greater ease.

Staying motivated for lifelong success is about nurturing a commitment that grows and adapts with you. It's the steady determination to keep making choices that align with your well-being, knowing that each day is another opportunity to build the life you envision. With every goal achieved, every new habit formed and every small step taken, you're creating a lasting foundation for health and happiness.

BONUS

✦

Welcome to the bonus page!
Here you can download the unmissable and beautiful **"30-Day Motivation Guide"**, your faithful ally in your post-surgery recovery journey.
Download it now!

SCAN THIS QR-CODE TO DOWNLOAD YOUR GREAT BONUS!

OR COPY AND PASTE THIS URL:
https://www.subscribepage.com/z7m6z2_copy10_copy2

Made in the USA
Las Vegas, NV
30 December 2024